西安交通大学 本科"十四五"规划教材 | 援外医疗队医学英语培训用书

主审 白永权 聂文信

临床医学英语阅读

Selected Readings in Clinical Medicine

主　编　李小棉　詹菊红

副主编　何宗昌　张桂梅　胡　滨　薛英利

编　者　傅明明　黄玉秀　金柏岑　刘　华
　　　　田荣昌　铁　瑛　熊淋宵　张晓枚
　　　　张晓谦　赵　娜　郑　青　朱晓娟

U0303768

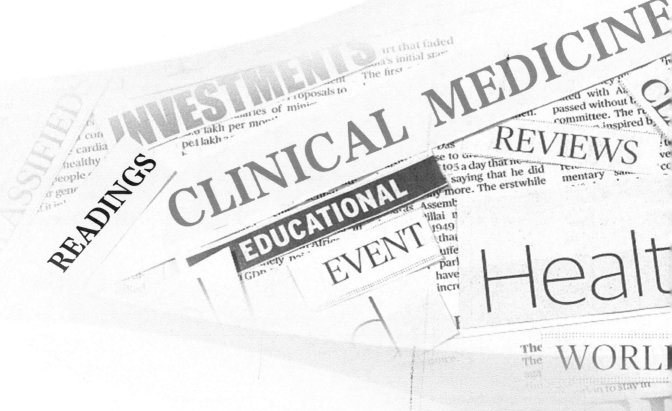

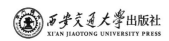

西安交通大学出版社
XI'AN JIAOTONG UNIVERSITY PRESS

图书在版编目(CIP)数据

临床医学英语阅读 / 李小棉,詹菊红主编. —西安:西安交通大学出版社,2022.5(2024.9 重印)
ISBN 978-7-5693-2551-5

Ⅰ.①临… Ⅱ.①李… ②詹… Ⅲ.①医学—英语—阅读教学—教材 Ⅳ.①R

中国版本图书馆 CIP 数据核字(2022)第 034365 号

书　　名	临床医学英语阅读	
	LINCHUANG YIXUE YINGYU YUEDU	
主　　编	李小棉　詹菊红	
责任编辑	庞钧颖　蔡乐芊	
责任校对	李　蕊	
封面设计	任加盟	
出版发行	西安交通大学出版社	
	(西安市兴庆南路 1 号　邮政编码 710048)	
网　　址	http://www.xjtupress.com	
电　　话	(029)82668357　82667874(市场营销中心)	
	(029)82668315(总编办)	
传　　真	(029)82668280	
印　　刷	西安五星印刷有限公司	
开　　本	850 mm×1168 mm　1/16　　印张　16.25　　字数　352 千字	
版次印次	2022 年 5 月第 1 版　　2024 年 9 月第 2 次印刷	
书　　号	ISBN 978-7-5693-2551-5	
定　　价	79.00 元	

如发现印装质量问题,请与本社市场营销中心联系。
订购热线:(029)82665248　(029)82667874
投稿热线:(029)82665371
读者信箱:xjtu_rw@163.com

前言

Preface

一、编写背景

医学英语课程是医学生培养方案中非常重要的一个部分。开设医学英语课程对于医学生的学习和未来职业发展大有裨益。作为国内医学英语教育研究基地，西安交通大学率先试点，为临床医学专业学生定制医学英语课程，包括医学英语词汇学、医学英语视听说、医学英语基础阅读、临床医学英语阅读和医学英语写作等课程内容，力求为医学生后续学习复杂的医学知识构建一个全面而坚实的医学英语语言框架，为本科三年级的临床医学课程提前打好医学英语语言基础。

目前，针对医学英语词汇学、医学英语视听说及医学英语基础阅读等课程，国内已有比较成熟的教材，而临床医学英语阅读方面的教材，却比较少见。历经两年半的时间，西安交通大学医学英语教学团队与全国医学英语专家及各大医学院校同仁倾力合作，完成了本教材的编写工作。

本教材既适合本科高年级医学英语课程，也可以作为医学院校研究生、博士生医学英语课程的配套教材。对于广大医务工作者来说，本教材也可作为自学或者阅读材料。

二、内容设计

全书共17章。每章均包括精读和泛读两部分。精读部分所选文章均来自国际权威期刊。泛读部分的内容涉及医学人文精神传承、医学技术革新、医学发展前沿探索等多个主题。

从题型设计来看，精读部分的练习包括8道大题，题目设置的主要目的是训练学生在字、词、句、篇等层面全方位提升专业英语的水平。第1题和第2题，针对阅读理解内容,从不同层面考查学生对所学疾病病原、病机、诊断、治疗和预防等方面相关内容的表达。第3题是关于疾病的简要综述,用回填重点词汇的方式让学生回顾疾病相关医学术语。第4题是医学英语句型训练,从所选文章中摘出常见医学英语表达句型,学生按照要求替换相应部分,使用黑体词汇进行造句,所造句子应和医学内容相关,重点练习医学英语表达句型。第5题是搭配题,要求学生把所列句子按所属医学主题归类,从而加深学生对各医学主题内容的了解。第6题包含2道小题:第1小题给出此类型段落发展方式的概念,该题要求学生根据概念标出所给段落的段落发展方式要素;第2小题是排序题,通过段落句子顺序重排训练,学生可进一步学习段落发展方式的要素及其应用。在段落发展方式练习中,所提供的段落内容皆与本章精读部分中所描述的疾病相关。第7题是翻译题,题目是关于本章节所讲疾病内容的中文综述,该题要求学生运用本节所学内容把中文内容翻译成英文,从而复习巩固所学内容。第8题设置阅读表格(预习、复习均可使用),包括词汇摘析、句子摘析、段落结构分析等项目。

泛读部分的练习设置旨在通过思政课程的内容,培养医学生高尚的大医情怀、严谨的治学态度和孜孜不倦的科研探索精神。

三、教学建议

第一、针对课前预习,教师可安排学生课前完成练习题第8题的阅读表格,让学生初步了解医学英语的语言特点。

第二、在课堂教学过程中,教师可把学生分组。助教收集每组的表格并对其进行批阅,总结出表格各个模块的完成情况,填写课前预习总结(见 Appendix 2)。教师可根据课前预习表格总结及学生的实际预习情况进行课堂设计。

在第一学时,建议进行以下教学安排。

(1)选择优秀组进行预习展示(约15分钟),然后对学生展示及预习情况当堂回馈(约25分钟),并讲解其他组的预习情况(约10分钟)。

(2)把2个预习小组合并为1个大组,各小组拿出自己的阅读表格,按照表格内容逐一进行互相讲评(约15分钟),完成后各组在班级进行汇报(约20分钟)。教师根据预习作业中的漏洞进行重点讲解(约15分钟)。

在第二学时,教师可根据班级情况自行安排,也可参考以下两种计划。

(1)指导学生列出某一词汇链并进行分析(约15分钟),词汇链可以是与疾病相关的医学词汇链,也可是文中某一部分的动词链、副词链等;指导学生分析某一种语法现象(约15分钟),如文中某一部分时态变化的情况,或标点符号使用情况等;指导学生学习典型句型(约20分钟)。

（2）指导学生进行语篇分析（约15分钟），如指导学生制作思维导图，分析文章结构，学习文中典型段落的发展方式等；教师讲解医学英语特点（约15分钟）；指导学生学习医学语言特点（约10分钟）；指导学生快速阅读泛读文章，辨析讨论相关的思政话题（约10分钟）。

第三，在课后复习过程中，教师可针对教学情况，安排相应的课后练习题目，并让学生重新整理阅读表格，巩固教学效果。

上述教学计划仅为参考。具体的课时安排和课程进度，各位教师可根据学校安排及个人情况进行调整。

最后，非常感谢西安交通大学和西安医学院援外项目对于本教材的大力支持！特别感谢西安交通大学外国语学院学术委员会的各位专家给教材提出的宝贵建议！尽管如此，教材难免会有纰漏之处，欢迎各位专家和同仁指正！

目 录

Contents

UNIT 1 Pneumatology

Respiratory disease affects one in five people and is the third leading cause of death in the world (after cancer and cardiovascular disease). Lung cancer, pneumonia and chronic obstructive pulmonary disease are the biggest causes of death in respiratory diseases.

Part I Intensive Reading

Chronic Obstructive Pulmonary Disease

Chronic obstructive pulmonary disease (COPD) is a common preventable and treatable disease characterized by persistent airflow limitation that is usually progressive and associated with an enhanced chronic inflammatory response in the airways and the lungs to harmful particles or gases.

Epidemiology

COPD is a major global health issue that is increasing in importance as a cause of death. The disease is currently the third leading cause of death worldwide, is ranked fifth in terms of disease burden, is greatly underdiagnosed, and is often diagnosed late in its course.

Most deaths from COPD occur in East and South Asia as this is where the largest proportion of world's population lives, These two regions also have the highest age-standardized mortality rates from COPD. What's more, COPD mortality rates are higher in men than in women and rise exponentially with age. It is the aging of the world's population over the past 20 years that has had the most influence on changing the relative importance of COPD as a cause of death.

By far the most common cause of chronic airflow obstruction globally is smoking and exposure to environmental tobacco smoke. The next most potent risk factor is a history of tuberculosis. In addition, the dust work environments, poverty, and lack of education also have their roles in COPD development.

Mechanisms/Pathophysiology

Not all cigarette smokers develop airway obstruction, indicating that there are susceptibility mechanisms—which might include genetic, epigenetic and environmental factors—that are currently poorly understood.

- Genetic risk factors

COPD tends to cluster in families and twin studies, pedigree studies, and analysis of unrelated individuals have all suggested that there is significant heritability of COPD, accounting for at least 30% of the variation in COPD risk. First-degree relatives of patients with COPD who smoke cigarettes have about a threefold increased risk of developing COPD compared with smokers from the general population.

- Pathogenesis

Pathology. The main pathological features of COPD are obstructive bronchiolitis, emphysema and, in many cases, mucus hypersecretion (chronic bronchitis), but the relative contribution of each of these pathologies to COPD varies between patients.

Chronic inflammation. COPD is associated with chronic inflammation that predominantly affects peripheral airways and lung parenchyma, although large airways also show inflammatory changes. The degree of inflammation increases with increased numbers of neutrophils, macrophages and lymphocytes in the lungs as the disease progresses.

Accelerated aging. COPD is largely a disease of the elderly and there is increasing evidence to indicate that emphysema is caused by accelerated aging of the lung parenchyma owing to defective endogenous anti-aging mechanisms with the activation of pathways leading to cellular senescence.

Oxidative stress. Increased oxidative stress is a key driving mechanism in the pathophysiology of COPD and accounts for many of the features of the disease.

Pathophysiology. The airway obstruction in COPD is predominantly in the small airways of the lung edge and results in a reduction in FEV_1 (Forced expiratory volume in 1 second) and the FEV_1/FVC (functional residual capacity) ratio, which progresses over time.

- Causes and pathogenesis of exacerbations

COPD exacerbations are episodes of symptom worsening that are usually associated with increased airway inflammation and systemic inflammatory effects. Most COPD exacerbations are triggered by respiratory viral infections, especially rhinovirus, which is the cause of the common cold and thus more common in winter.

Diagnosis

The diagnosis of COPD should be suspected in individuals with respiratory symptoms, such as cough, expectoration of sputum, shortness of breath upon exertion or lower respiratory tract infections occurring more frequently or lasting longer than expected (>2 weeks). The suspicion should increase if the individuals also report risk factors for COPD, such as exposure to cigarette smoke, environmental or occupational pollutants and/or the presence of a family history of obstructive lung diseases.

History of exposure to risk factors. The most important risk factors for COPD are the inhalation of particulate matter from cigarette smoke and the burning of biomass for cooking or heating. Other risk factors for COPD development include second-hand exposure to cigarette smoke or other particulate matter during infancy, socioeconomic disadvantage, childhood respiratory symptoms, and asthma during the growth period.

Clinical presentation. Most individuals with mild disease have a normal physical examination, including pulse, respiratory rate, chest expansion, and breath and heart sounds. However, the use of a standardized functional grading of dyspnea, the most important symptom of respiratory compromise, can help to increase the degree of suspicion, direct the health care provider to implement a spirometry test and help to stage disease severity.

One such scale is the Modified Medical Research Council Dyspnea Scale, graded from 0 to 4 with the lowest grade implying no dyspnea with any activity and the highest grade implying dyspnea with minimal activity. In patients with more-advanced disease, increased respiratory rate with forced expiratory efforts, decreased breath sounds on chest auscultation, the presence of rhonchi, coarse crackles, and wheezes and, in the most advanced cases, cyanosis (blue skin discoloration, a sign of hypoxemia) might be present and should be considered an important complication that requires therapy with oxygen.

Currently, the non-invasive pulse oximetry enables the determination of hypoxemia early and oxygen should be prescribed for patients with saturations below 88% while breathing room air. The failure of the right heart due to hypoxemia and increased intrapulmonary vascular resistance is characterized by severe dyspnea, impaired exercise capacity, leg edema and, in the most severe cases, generalized edema.

COPD is a complex heterogeneous disease in which the majority of patients combine features of the classic subgroups of the "pink puffer" and the "blue bloater" phenotypes. Pink puffers have lower muscle mass, more emphysema, and fewer cardiovascular and metabolic co-morbidities than blue bloaters who have higher body mass index with less emphysema and more metabolic co-morbidities and cardiac compromise.

Confirming the diagnosis. A diagnosis of COPD is confirmed by the documentation of expiratory airflow limitation during a forced expiratory maneuver from total lung capacity to residual volume. This measurement is easily achieved using a simple spirometer and recording the timed FVC following standard recommendations. Many patients, and more so in advanced disease stages, will have increased lung volumes and air trapping that are measured by body plethysmography using a sealed body box.

Global assessment and co-morbidities. In acknowledgement of the multiple dimensions of COPD, several proposals for its comprehensive assessment have been developed. The most widely evaluated of these assessments is the body mass index, degree of obstruction, dyspnea, and exercise capacity (BODE) index and its variants, such as the BODEx (in which the exercise is substituted by the rate of exacerbations). Other assessments include the age, dyspnea and obstruction (ADO) index, and the dyspnea, obstruction, smoking and exacerbation (DOSE) index.

Several co-morbidities also occur more frequently in patients with COPD than in patients without the disease and increase the risk of death. These co-morbidities include coronary artery disease, arrhythmias including tachycardia, hypertension, and congestive heart failure. Of particular importance are the increased risks of lung cancer, depression and anxiety, metabolic syndrome and osteoporosis.

Imaging. A chest X-ray helps eliminate other diagnoses, such as interstitial lung diseases, congestive heart failure, pleural effusions, and most pulmonary infections. CT scanning can estimate the degree of emphysema and its distribution and identify bronchial wall thickening, bronchiectasis (widening of the airway) and gas trapping (on expiration views).

Management

- Stable disease

    Management of stable (non-exacerbating) disease can be divided into the following categories: reducing exposure to harmful substances, relief of symptoms and reducing risk, mainly the risk of exacerbations.

    Non-pharmacological treatment. Pulmonary rehabilitation can be defined as an interdisciplinary program of care for patients with chronic respiratory impairment that is individually tailored and designed to optimize each patient's physical and social performance and autonomy. Programs comprise individualized exercise programs and education.

    Pharmacological treatment. Treatment with bronchodilators is the mainstay of pharmacological management of symptoms and primarily addresses breathlessness. Bronchodilators include β2-agonists and muscarinic receptor antagonists (anticholinergics). Inhaled long-acting bronchodilators of 12 – 24 hours of duration are preferred and, of these, long-acting β2-agonists (LABAs) and long-acting muscarinic antagonists (LAMAs) are equally effective. Patients with a history of exacerbations and/or low lung function are at particular risk of future exacerbations. Several drug classes reduce the risk of exacerbations, including long-acting bronchodilators, inhaled corticosteroids (ICSs), macrolides, phosphodiesterase type 4 (PDE4) inhibitors and mucolytics. Adverse effects are mainly limited to dryness of the mouth for anticholinergics, and tremor and hypokalemia for β2-agonists.

    Surgical intervention. Lung volume reduction surgery and transplantation are evidence-based interventions that can improve survival and quality of life in highly selected patients, usually those with very severe disease.

- Exacerbations

    COPD exacerbations are defined in the GOLD (Global Initiative for Chronic Obstructive Lung Disease) strategy in terms of health care utilization as "an acute event characterized by a worsening of the patient's respiratory symptoms that is beyond normal day-to-day variations and leads to a change in medication". The main symptoms of a COPD exacerbation are increases in dyspnea, sputum purulence and cough, but other symptoms might include increased wheezing and symptoms of a cold. COPD exacerbations are a major cause of admissions and readmissions to hospital and are also independent predictors of mortality in COPD.

    Pharmacological treatment. Management of an exacerbation comprises oral antibiotics, such as amoxicillin, if there is evidence of increased sputum purulence or volume. The choice of antibiotic will depend on the patient's history and underlying disease severity. Oral corticosteroids in short courses are also added, depending on the individual exacerbation severity.

Exacerbation prevention. Usual treatments decrease exacerbation frequency and improve quality of life in patients with COPD. These treatments include influenza vaccination, use of long-acting bronchodilators, LAMAs, antibiotics, azithromycin, mucolytic drugs, and performing pulmonary rehabilitation etc. However, significant rates of hearing decrement (as measured by audiometry) and antibiotic resistance were reported for azithromycin use.

Quality of Life

Patients with COPD report an impaired health status, irrespective of the severity of the disease. An improvement in health status is associated with starting polymedication, pulmonology visits, balanced diet, completing a rehabilitation program, smoking cessation and a reduction in the number of exacerbations. By contrast, a decline in health status is associated with worsening respiratory symptoms and increased hospitalizations. This bidirectional association underlines the importance of the routine monitoring of health status in these patients.

Owing to the systemic effects of the disease, one study found that 97.7% of patients with COPD had one or more comorbidity and 53.5% were diagnosed with four or more co-morbidities. Each additional comorbidity increases the chance of worsening of self-rated health by 43%. Unfortunately, comorbidities are often underdiagnosed and consequently under-treated, which might consequently worsen COPD prognosis.

Prevention

The most effective way to combat the worldwide epidemic of COPD is the implementation of social, economic and educational programs aimed at decreasing the uptake of cigarette smoking. This primary prevention effort should be particularly aimed at teenagers, as this is the group in which addiction begins and is the target of large tobacco corporations. The other considerable risk factor that can be controlled is that of exposure to biomass combustion particles. Thus, improvement in working environments and living conditions and diet might also be efficacious.

(Extracted from *Nature*)

Vocabulary

exponentially	[ˌekspə'nenʃəlɪ]	*adv*. 成倍地;指数地
epigenetic	[ˌepɪdʒɪ'netɪk]	*adj*. 外成的;后成的
pedigree	['pedɪgriː]	*n*. 家谱;系谱;血统
parenchyma	[pə'reŋkɪmə]	*n*. 实质
senescence	[sɪ'nesns]	*n*. 衰老
oxidative	['ɒksɪdeɪtɪv]	*adj*. 氧化的
rhinovirus	[ˌraɪnəʊ'vaɪərəs]	*n*. 鼻病毒
expectoration	[ɪkˌspektə'reɪʃn]	*n*. 咳痰;吐痰;吐出物
compromise	['kɒmprəmaɪz]	*n*. 损伤
spirometry	[spaɪə'rɒmɪtrɪ]	*n*. 肺活量测定法
auscultation	[ˌɔːskəl'teɪʃn]	*n*. 听诊
rhonchi	['rɒŋkɪ]	*n*. (rhonchus 的复数)干啰音
cyanosis	[ˌsaɪə'nəʊsɪs]	*n*. 紫绀
oximetry	[ɒk'sɪmɪtrɪ]	*n*. 血氧定量法
saturation	[ˌsætʃə'reɪʃn]	*n*. 饱和;饱和度;浸透
heterogeneous	[ˌhetərə'dʒiːnɪəs]	*adj*. 异种的;异质的
phenotype	['fiːnətaɪp]	*n*. 显型;表现型
maneuver	[mə'nuːvə]	*n*. 方法
spirometer	[ˌspaɪ'rɒmɪtə]	*n*. 肺活量计
plethysmography	[pliθɪz'mɒgrəfɪ]	*n*. 体积描记术
effusion	[ɪ'fjuːʒn]	*n*. 流出;溢出
interdisciplinary	[ˌɪntə'dɪsəplɪnərɪ]	*adj*. 跨学科的
agonist	['ægənɪst]	*n*. 收缩筋;兴奋剂
muscarinic	[ˌmʌskə'rɪnɪk]	*adj*. 毒蕈碱的
antagonist	[æn'tægənɪst]	*n*. 对抗剂;拮抗剂
anticholinergics	[ˌæntɪˌkɒlɪ'nɜːdʒɪks]	*n*. 抗胆碱能药物
corticosteroid	[ˌkɔːtɪkəʊ'steərɔɪd]	*n*. 皮质类固醇
macrolide	['mækrəlaɪd]	*n*. 大环内酯物
phosphodiesterase	[fɒsfədaɪə'stereɪs]	*n*. 磷酸二酯酶
inhibitor	[ɪn'hɪbɪtə(r)]	*n*. 抑制物
mucolytic	[ˌmjuːkəʊ'lɪtɪk]	*adj*. 黏液溶解的
purulence	['pjʊərʊləns]	*n*. 脓;化脓
amoxicillin	[ə'mɒksɪˌsɪlɪn]	*n*. 阿莫西林
azithromycin	[eɪzɪθrə'maɪsɪn]	*n*. 阿奇霉素

| decrement | [ˈdekrɪmənt] | n. 渐减；减少 |
| audiometry | [ˌɔːdɪˈɒmətrɪ] | n. 听觉测试法 |

Exercises

1. **Read the text and explain the following medical phrases.**

   1) Clinical characteristics of COPD
   2) Risk factors for the development of COPD
   3) Pathological features of COPD
   4) Guidelines to manage stable COPD
   5) Symptoms of COPD exacerbations

2. **Answer the following questions according to the text.**

   1) How can COPD be diagnosed and staged?
   2) What tests can be used to confirm COPD?
   3) What co-morbidities can occur in patients with COPD?
   4) How can COPD be prevented?

3. **Fill in the blanks with the proper forms of the given words.**

   > exposure   dyspnea   patient   decompensation   epidemiology
   > prevalence   underestimate   develop   present   suspect

   Not infrequently, and usually in more-advanced cases, COPD is suspected at the time of a severe respiratory 1) _____ due to an acute exacerbation or following surgeries, such as upper abdominal or thoracic procedures. This deterioration is caused by the main problem of underdiagnoses, as most individuals with the disease 2) _____ their symptoms, assuming that they are the natural consequence of a smoking habit, aging or job 3) _____ . Furthermore, even in moderate-to-advanced stages of COPD, the affected 4) _____ will become ever more sedentary to avoid the uncomfortable symptom of exertional 5) _____ . Unfortunately, many health care providers fail to consider a diagnosis of COPD in patients 6) _____ with these symptoms, especially if the person is a woman or relatively young. The reasons for the failure to 7) _____ COPD in these groups rests on older studies of the 8) _____ of COPD that described the disease as being one of older men. As the smoking habit has increased in younger individuals and the 9) _____ of COPD in women is now approaching or has surpassed（in some developed countries）that of men, COPD is now prevalent in younger individuals and particularly in women, who might actually (10) _____ the disease at an earlier age than men.

4. **Study the bold-faced words in each of the following sentences and imitate the particular way of writing.**

Mentor Sentence:

☆ In morbidly obese patients, bariatric surgery **can be an effective means of** weight loss.

Imitation Sentence:

☆ Parenteral vaccination **can be an effective means of** inducing protective mucosal responses.

1) **The main pathological features of** COPD **are** obstructive bronchiolitis, emphysema and, in many cases, mucus hypersecretion (chronic bronchitis).

Answer: **The main pathological features of** _____ **are** _____

_____

2) Increased oxidative stress **is a key driving mechanism in the pathophysiology of** COPD **and accounts for** many of the features of the disease.

Answer: _____ **is a key driving mechanism in the pathophysiology of** _____ **and accounts for** _____

3) Most COPD exacerbations **are triggered by** respiratory viral infections, especially rhinovirus, **which** is the cause of the common cold and thus more common in winter.

Answer: _____ **are/is triggered by** _____

_____ ,

which _____

4) **The main symptoms of** a COPD exacerbation **are** increases in dyspnea, sputum purulence and cough, **but other symptoms might include** increased wheezing and symptoms of a cold.

Answer: **The main symptoms of** _____ **are** _____ , **but other symptoms might include** _____

5. **Match the following statements with the corresponding sections in the text.**

Epidemiology: _____   Management: _____

Mechanisms/Pathophysiology: _____   Quality of Life: _____

Diagnosis: _____   Prevention: _____

A. Chronic obstructive pulmonary disease (COPD) is a common disease with high global morbidity and mortality.

B. COPD is characterized by poorly reversible airway obstruction, which is confirmed by spirometry, and includes obstruction of the small airways (chronic obstructive bronchiolitis) and emphysema, which lead to air trapping and shortness of breath in response to physical exertion.

C. The most common risk factor for the development of COPD is cigarette smoking, but other environmental factors, such as exposure to indoor air pollutants—especially in developing countries—might influence COPD risk.

D. Not all smokers develop COPD and the reasons for disease susceptibility in these individuals have not been fully elucidated.

E. Although the mechanisms underlying COPD remain poorly understood, the disease is associated with chronic inflammation that is usually corticosteroid resistant.

F. In addition, COPD involves accelerated aging of the lungs and an abnormal repair mechanism that might be driven by oxidative stress.

G. Acute exacerbations, which are mainly triggered by viral or bacterial infections, are important as they are linked to a poor prognosis.

H. The mainstay of the management of stable disease is the use of inhaled long-acting bronchodilators, whereas corticosteroids are beneficial primarily in patients who have coexisting features of asthma, such as eosinophilic inflammation and more reversibility of airway obstruction. Apart from smoking cessation, no treatments reduce disease progression.

I. More research is needed to better understand disease mechanisms and to develop new treatments that reduce disease activity and progression.

6. Read the introduction in the box and finish the exercises after it.

> In composition, **spatial order** is an organizational structure in which details are presented as they are (or were) located in space—from left to right, top to bottom, etc.

1) Draw a brief picture of the respiratory tract according to the description in the passage below.

The air that we breathe in enters the nose or mouth, flows through the throat (pharynx) and voice box (larynx) and enters the windpipe (trachea). The trachea divides into two hollow tubes called bronchi. The right main bronchus (bronchus is the word for one of the bronchi) supplies the right lung; the left main bronchus supplies the left lung. These bronchi then go on to divide into smaller bronchi. The small bronchi divide into smaller and smaller hollow tubes, which are called bronchioles—the smallest air tubes in the lungs. The medical term for all the air tubes from the nose and mouth down to the bronchioles is "the respiratory tract". The lower respiratory tract is from the larynx.

2) Reorder the following sentences to make an effective paragraph.

A. Beside and above the uppermost concha is the olfactory region of the nasal cavity.

B. The shape of the nasal cavity is complex.

C. The rest of the cavity is the respiratory portion.

D. The forward section, within and above each nostril, is called the vestibule.

E. Behind the vestibule and along each outer wall are three elevations, running generally from front to rear.

F. Sinus cavities are located in the bony skull on both sides of the nose.

G. The respiratory area is lined with a moist mucous membrane with fine hairlike projections known as cilia, which serve to collect debris.

H. Each elevation, called a nasal concha or turbinate, hangs over an air passage.

I. Mucus from cells in the membrane wall also helps to trap particles of dust, carbon, soot, and bacteria.

Answer： __ __ __ __ __ __ __ __ __

7. **Translate the Chinese paragraph below into English.**

　　慢性阻塞性肺病是以持续性气流受限为主要表现的呼吸道炎症性病变,随病情进展可引起肺组织结构和功能损害,并对患者身心健康和日常生活造成不利影响。其发病机制现阶段尚未完全明确,但空气污染、职业性粉尘及吸烟等是全世界公认的致病因素。

8. **Read the text and fill in the sheet with proper information.**

Reading Prompts	
Items	**Your Answers**
1) *Identify the medical terms concerning* **COPD** *and group them according to your understanding.*	
2) *Identify the* **adjectives** *used in* "**Clinical Presentation**" *and explain what conditions they describe.*	

continued

Reading Prompts	
Items	**Your Answers**
3) *Identify the **conjunctions** used in* **"Quality of Life"** *and point out the logical relation each of them indicates.*	
4) *Identify the **verbs** used in* **Exercise 3** *and point out the changes of verb tenses.*	
5) *Identify the **typical sentence patterns**.（**the whole article**）*	
6) *Identify the **topic sentence** and **the supporting sentences** in* **"Prevention"**.	

Part II Extensive Reading

Title: _____

Over two hundred years ago, an epochal work was published, which was to radically change the art of healing. *On Mediate Auscultation or Treatise on the Diagnosis of the Diseases of the Lungs and Heart* (translated from French)—928 pages in two volumes, was already celebrated as the "New Testament of Medicine" at that time. In 1823, the author was admitted to the Mount Olympus of French science as professor of the medical faculty of Paris and head of the Charité, and as chevalier of the Legion of Honor. By inventing the stethoscope, Théophile René Hyacinthe Laennëc had steered medicine towards carefully targeted analysis and precise diagnostics as opposed to the previously dominating form of medicine, which was based on guesswork and obscure theorems.

As his mother died early, presumably from pulmonary tuberculosis, Laënnec left Quimper and grew up at an uncle's home. During the revolutionary wars, he witnessed the besiegement of Nantes and the care for the wounded. Fascinated by medicine at an early age, he started his formal medical education at the age of 19 in Paris. Important personages, such as Dupuytren and Corvisart, Napoleon's personal physician, were among his teachers, and the latter instructed him in the almost forgotten art of percussion. Laënnec's fondness for music, especially for playing the flute, which he pursued with passion—including the occasional public performance at aristocrats' homes—was not without relevance in regard to his later discovery and interpretation of the auscultation results.

The actual invention of the stethoscope by Laënnec can be traced back to several inspirations. In December 1816, Laënnec observed two children in the park of the Louvre, who put their ears at the ends of a wooden bar and transmitted tapping signals to each other, which were acoustically amplified by the wood. According to Laënnec's own words, the clinical application of this observation emerged when he was consulted by a young woman who showed symptoms of a general cardiac disease. The age and gender of the patient prohibited him from placing his ear directly on her chest. Instead, he took a paper notebook, made it into a tight roll, placed one end on the heart region, and, putting his ear on the other end, he was as surprised as he was satisfied to hear the sequence of heartbeats much clearer and cleaner than it had ever been possible by a direct placement of the ear. The idea of the stethoscope was born! —Laënnec constructed a more solid version of the ear trumpet in the form of a wooden hollow cylinder of 25 cm length and 2.5 cm diameter, which, in a later variant, could be assembled from three parts. Laënnec used cedar or ebony wood and manufactured the stethoscope himself. He sold the stethoscopes at a low price together with his book, published in the first edition in 1819—a visionary anticipation of a marketing idea that can only be called shrewd in colloquial terms. The term stethoscope, by the way, is made up of the two Greek words, stethos, which means "chest" and skopein, that is "to see and observe". With the help of the new instrument, the examining physician was able to hear various breathing sounds, such as bronchial breathing, shoulder sounds, as well as heart tones, diastolic sounds and the galloping rhythm characteristic for mitral stenosis. Laënnec, together with Harvey and Senac, was thus among the first to describe atrial fibrillation, after he had noticed the variation of the heart contraction, with or without palpable pulse—in accordance with the modern definition of pulse deficit.

Laënnec's interpretation of the heart sounds S1 and S2 was not correct according to our current state of knowledge, but his discovery soon found worldwide use and recognition. Nevertheless, his scientific and pathophysiological ideas did not remain uncontested. Broussais in particular, a well-known physician also hailing from Brittany, attacked Laënnec sharply to the point of personal denigration and public defamation, which was then returned in kind by Laënnec. Interestingly enough, great French hospitals today carry the name of both rivals of old. Despite all animosities, Laënnec gained increasingly in prestige and esteem. He auscultated the chest of Madame de Staël as well as that of Chateaubriand and various cardinals.

Laënnec was a Breton with heart and soul. He loved the country and its people; he spoke their (Breton) language as well as Latin and Greek and the world languages Italian, English, and German; French, of course. He had a close relationship with the church. Laënnec was again and again drawn back to his native region, where he enjoyed the fresh air on extended hikes, which later also helped to alleviate his tuberculosis-caused symptoms. Brittany, i.e. his house Kerlouarnec, was also the place to which Laënnec withdrew when he felt that the end of his life was near. On 9 June 1826, he believed to have only one week left to live. In reality, he died on 13 August 1826, from pulmonary tuberculosis, the disease, to the diagnosis of which he had contributed so tremendously. Laënnec died highly venerated and now on his former house of birth stand plaques to commemorate his contribution to medicine.

(Extracted from https://link springer.com)

Exercises

1. Read the article and write a possible title for it.

2. Answer the following questions according to the passage.

    1）How significant is the invention of stethoscope?

    2）What talent has promoted Laënnec to invent stethoscope?

    3）What cases have enhanced the inspiration of inventing stethoscope?

    4）How is stethoscope named?

    5）What personalities had made Laënnec successful?

UNIT 2 Obstetrics and Gynecology

Obstetrics and gynecology is the medical specialty that encompasses the two subspecialties of obstetrics (covering pregnancy, childbirth, and the postpartum period) and gynecology (covering the health of the female reproductive system— vagina, uterus, ovaries, and breasts). The diseases of obstetrics and gynecology include menstrual disorders, preeclampsia, uterine fibroids, endometriosis and vaginal discharge etc.

Part I Intensive Reading

Preeclampsia

Preeclampsia (PE) is a disorder of pregnancy associated with new-onset hypertension, which occurs most often after 20 weeks of gestation and frequently near term. Although often accompanied by new onset proteinuria, hypertension and other signs or symptoms, some women with preeclampsia may not present proteinuria. Other than the delivery of the fetus and the removal of the placenta, to date there are no therapeutic approaches to treat or prevent PE. It is thus only possible to reduce PE-related mortality through early detection, careful monitoring, and treatment of the symptoms.

Epidemiology

Hypertensive disorders of pregnancy constitute one of the leading causes of maternal and perinatal mortality worldwide. It has been estimated that preeclampsia complicates 2%–8% of pregnancies globally. In Latin America and the Caribbean, hypertensive disorders are responsible for almost 26% of maternal deaths, whereas in Africa and Asia they contribute to 9% of deaths. Although maternal mortality is much lower in high-income countries than in developing countries, 16% of maternal deaths can be attributed to hypertensive disorders. In the United States, the rate of preeclampsia increased by 25% between 1987 and 2004. Moreover, in comparison with women giving birth in 1980, those giving birth in 2003 were at 6.7-fold increased risk of severe preeclampsia.

Several risk factors for the development of preeclampsia have been identified. The risk to the fetus in patients with preeclampsia relates largely to the gestational age at delivery. Risk to the mother can be significant and includes the possible development of disseminated intravascular coagulation, intracranial hemorrhage, renal failure, retinal detachment, pulmonary edema, liver rupture, abruptio placentae, and even death. Therefore, astute and experienced clinicians should be caring for women with preeclampsia.

Mechanisms/Pathophysiology

The etiology of preeclampsia remains unknown. During the past century, many theories regarding its etiology have been suggested, but most have not withstood the test of time. The syndrome is characterized by vasospasm, hemoconcentration, and ischemic changes in the placenta, kidney, liver and brain. These syndromes are usually seen in women with severe preeclampsia. Theories as to the causative mechanisms include placental origin, immunologic origin, and genetic predisposition among others. A great deal of research is dedicated to solving the etiologic enigma of preeclampsia. Without a definitive etiology, predicting patients at risk for the development of preeclampsia and effecting a treatment are difficult.

- Vascular

The hypertensive changes seen in preeclampsia are attributed to intense vasospasm thought to be caused by increased vascular reactivity. The underlying mechanism responsible for the increased vascular reactivity is presumed to be alterations in the normal interactions of vasodilatory (prostacyclin and nitric oxide) and vasoconstrictive (thromboxane A2 and endothelin) substances. Another vascular hallmark of preeclampsia is hemoconcentration. Patients with preeclampsia have lower intravascular volumes and have less tolerance for the blood loss associated with delivery.

- Hematologic

The most common hematologic abnormality in preeclampsia is thrombocytopenia (platelet count less than $100,000/mm^3$). The exact mechanism for thrombocytopenia is unknown. Another possible hematologic abnormality is microangiopathic hemolysis as seen in association with HELLP syndrome and can be diagnosed by schistocytes seen on peripheral smear and increased lactate dehydrogenase (LDH) levels. Interpretation of the baseline hematocrit level in a preeclamptic patient may be difficult. A low hematocrit level may signify hemolysis and a falsely high hematocrit may be caused by hemoconcentration.

- Hepatic changes

Hepatic damage in association with preeclampsia can range from mildly elevated liver enzyme levels to subcapsular liver hematomas and hepatic ruptures. The latter are usually associated with HELLP syndrome. The pathologic liver lesions seen on autopsy are periportal hemorrhages, ischemic lesions, and fibrin deposition.

- Renal changes

Vasospasm in preeclampsia leads to decreased renal perfusion and subsequent decreased "glomerular filtration rate" (GFR). In normal pregnancy the GFR is increased up to 50% above prepregnancy levels. Because of this, serum creatinine levels in preeclamptic patients rarely increase above normal pregnancy levels (0.8 mg/dL). Close monitoring of urine output is necessary in patients with preeclampsia, because oliguria (defined as less than 500 cc/24 hours) may occur because of renal insufficiency. Rarely, profound renal insufficiency may lead to acute tubular necrosis. The pathognomonic renal lesion in preeclampsia is called glomerular capillary endotheliosis, which is swelling of the glomerular capillary endothelial and mesangial cells.

- Central nervous system

Eclamptic convulsions are perhaps the most disturbing central nervous system (CNS) manifestation of preeclampsia and remain a major cause of maternal mortality in the developing countries. The exact etiology of eclampsia is unknown but is thought to be attributed to hypertensive encephalopathy and vasospasm with resultant ischemia or microhemorrhages and cerebral edema. Radiologic studies may show evidence of cerebral edema and hemorrhagic lesions, particularly in the posterior hemispheres, which may explain the visual disturbances seen in preeclampsia. Other CNS abnormalities include headaches and visual disturbances such as scotomata, photophobia, blurred vision, and, rarely, temporary blindness.

- Fetus and placenta

The hallmark placental lesion in preeclampsia is acute atherosclerosis of the decidual arteries. This is caused in part by the abnormal adaptation of the spiral artery/cytotrophoblast interface and results in poor perfusion. This may lead to poor placental perfusion, resulting in oligohydramnios, intrauterine growth restriction, placental abruption fetal distress, and, ultimately, fetal demise.

Diagnosis

- Gestational hypertension

Gestational hypertension is defined as a systolic blood pressure of 140 mmHg or more or a diastolic blood pressure of 90 mmHg or more, or both, on two occasions at least 4 hours apart after 20 weeks of gestation in a woman with a previously normal blood pressure. Women with gestational hypertension with severe range blood pressures (a systolic blood pressure of 160 mmHg or higher, or diastolic blood pressure of 110 mmHg or higher) should be diagnosed with preeclampsia with severe features.

- Preeclampsia

The rate of preeclampsia ranges between 2% and 7% in healthy nulliparous women. The rate is substantially higher in women with twin gestation (14%) and those with previous preeclampsia (18%). Preeclampsia is primarily defined as gestational hypertension plus proteinuria (300 mg/24 hours). If a 24-hour urine collection is not available, then proteinuria is defined as a concentration of 30mg/dL or more ($\geqslant$1+ on dipstick) in at least two random urine samples collected at least 6 hours apart. The urine dipstick measurements used to establish proteinuria should be no more than 7 days apart. Preeclampsia may be further subdivided into mild and severe forms. The distinction between the two is made on the basis of the degree of hypertension, proteinuria, and the involvement of other organ systems. The criteria for mild preeclampsia and severe preeclampsia are presented in Table 1.

Table 1 Classification of Preeclampsia

Mild Preeclampsia	Severe Preeclampsia
Blood pressure$\geqslant$140/90—2 occasions 6 h apart (not more than 1 week apart)	Blood Pressure$\geqslant$160/110—2 occasions at least 6 h apart (not more than 1 week apart)
Proteinuria—$\geqslant$300mg/24-h sample	Proteinuria—$\geqslant$5g/24-h sample
Or	Or

Mild Preeclampsia	Severe Preeclampsia
≥1+on 2 urine samples 6 h apart (not more than 1 week apart)	≥3+on 2 urine samples 6 h apart (not more than 1 week)
	Oliguria—<500mL/24 h
	Thrombocytopenia—<100,000/mm^3
	Epigastric or right upper quadrant pain
	Pulmonary edema
	Persistent cerebral or visual disturbances

In the absence of proteinuria, preeclampsia should be considered when gestational hypertension is associated with persistent cerebral symptoms, epigastric or right upper quadrant pain with nausea or vomiting, or in association with thrombocytopenia and abnormal liver enzymes.

Close surveillance of patients with either mild or severe preeclampsia is warranted because either type may progress to fulminant disease. A particularly severe form of preeclampsia is the HELLP syndrome, which is an acronym for hemolysis (H), elevated liver enzymes (EL), and low platelet count (LP). This syndrome is manifest by laboratory findings consistent with hemolysis, elevated levels of liver function tests, and thrombocytopenia. The diagnosis may be deceptive because blood pressure measurements may be only marginally elevated. A patient with HELLP syndrome is automatically classified as having severe preeclampsia. Another severe form of preeclampsia is eclampsia, which is the occurrence of seizures not attributable to other causes.

Management

- Delivery versus expectant management

At the initial evaluation, a complete blood count with platelet estimate, serum creatinine, LDH, AST, ALT, and testing for proteinuria should be obtained in parallel with a comprehensive clinical maternal and fetal evaluation.

In the settings of diagnostic dilemmas, such as in the evaluation of possible preeclampsia superimposed upon chronic hypertension, a uric acid test may be considered. Fetal evaluation should include ultrasonographic evaluation for estimated fetal weight, amount of amniotic fluid, and fetal antepartum testing. Subsequent management will depend on the results of the evaluation and gestational age. The decision to deliver must balance the maternal and fetal risks.

Preeclampsia with severe features can result in acute and long-term complications for the woman and her newborn. Maternal complications include pulmonary edema, myocardial infarction, stroke, acute respiratory distress syndrome, coagulopathy, renal failure, and retinal injury. These complications are more likely to occur in the presence of preexistent medical disorders. The clinical course of preeclampsia with severe features is characterized by progressive deterioration of maternal and fetal condition. Therefore, delivery is recommended when gestational hypertension or preeclampsia with severe features is diagnosed at or beyond 34 0/7 weeks of gestation, after maternal stabilization or with labor or pre-labor rupture of membranes. Delivery should not be delayed for the administration of steroids will be performed in the late preterm period.

- Inpatient versus outpatient management

Ambulatory management at home is an option only for women with gestational hypertension or preeclampsia without severe features but they are required to have frequent fetal and maternal evaluation. Hospitalization is appropriate for women with severe features and for women in whom adherence to frequent monitoring is a concern. Since assessment of blood pressure is essential for this clinical condition, and health care providers are encouraged to follow the recommendations from regulatory organizations regarding the proper technique for blood pressure measurement.

- Intrapartum management

In addition to appropriate management of labor and delivery, the two main goals of management of women with preeclampsia during labor and delivery are prevention of seizures and control of hypertension.

Quality of Life

Physical and mental wellbeing of women with a history of severe preeclampsia seems to be impaired. Sufficient support for this group of women is needed. This can provide a lot of help for their postpartum return to normal life. Obstetric caregivers should be aware of poor health-related quality of life, particularly mental health quality of life in women who have experienced severe preeclampsia (especially those confronted with perinatal death or their child's admission to a neonatal intensive care unit) and should consider referring the patients to postpartum psychological care.

Prevention

Although our understanding of etiology is still limited, the possibility of detecting and evaluating certain angiogenic factors by the end of the first trimester gives prospects for preeclampsia prevention. Secondary prevention is currently based mostly on the effort to pharmacologically affect the spiral artery transformation and the development of the abnormal placental microcirculation which lead to clinical symptoms of preeclampsia. Calcium supplementation is effective only in women with low calcium intake.

(Extracted from https//www. tchc. org)

Vocabulary

preeclampsia	[ˌpriːˈklæmpsɪə]	n. 先兆子痫
angiogenic	[ˌændʒɪəʊˈdʒenɪk]	adj. 生成血管的
eclampsia	[ɪˈklæmpsɪə]	n. 子痫
hemoconcentration	[heməkɒnsənˈtreɪʃn]	n. 血浓缩
prostacyclin	[ˌprɒstəˈsaɪklɪn]	n. 环前列腺素
thromboxane	[θrɒmˈbɒkseɪn]	n. 血栓素
endothelin	[endɒˈθiːlɪn]	n. 内皮素
thrombocytopenia	[ˌθrɒmbə(ʊ)ˌsaɪtə(ʊ)ˈpiːnɪə]	n. 血小板减少(症)
hemolysis	[hiːˈmɒlɪsɪs]	n. 溶血(现象)
glomerular	[glɒˈmerʊlə(r)]	adj. 肾小球的
vacuolated	[ˈvækjʊəleɪtɪd]	adj. 有液泡的
proteinuria	[ˌprəʊtiːˈnjʊərɪə]	n. 蛋白尿
nulliparous	[nʌˈlɪpərəs]	adj. 未生育过的
serum	[ˈsɪərəm]	n. 血清
creatinine	[kriːˈætəˌniːn]	n. 肌酸酐
expectant	[ɪkˈspektənt]	adj. 怀孕的;待产的
antepartum	[ˌæntɪˈpɑːtəm]	adj. 产前的;分娩前的
intrapartum	[ˌɪntrəˈpɑːtəm]	adj. 分娩期的

Exercises

1. Read the text and explain the following medical phrases.

1) Definition for preeclampsia

2) Vascular changes in women with preeclampsia

3) Hematologic changes in women with preeclampsia

4) Hepatic changes in women with preeclampsia

5) Renal changes in women with preeclampsia

2. Answer the following questions according to the article.

1) What are the classical criteria to diagnose preeclampsia?

2) What does HELLP syndrome mean?

3) Why is it important to treat women with preeclampsia during delivery?

4) When should the woman with preeclampsia be hospitalized?

3. Fill in the blanks with the proper forms of the given words.

delivery	complication	acute	rupture	infarction
deteriorate	edema	diagnose	syndrome	failure

Preeclampsia with severe features can result in 1) _____ and long-term complications for the woman and her newborn. Maternal complications include pulmonary 2) _____, myocardial 3) _____, stroke, acute respiratory distress 4)_____, coagulopathy, renal 5)_____, and retinal injury. These 6) _____ are more likely to occur in the presence of preexistent medical disorders. The clinical course of preeclampsia with severe features is characterized by progressive 7)_____ of maternal and fetal condition. Therefore, 8)_____ is recommended when gestational hypertension or preeclampsia with severe features is 9)_____ at or beyond 34 0/7 weeks of gestation, after maternal stabilization or with labor or prelabor 10) _____ of membranes. Delivery should not be delayed for the administration of steroids in the late preterm period.

4. Study the bold-faced words in each of the following sentences and imitate the particular way of writing.

Mentor Sentence:

☆ In morbidly obese patients, bariatric surgery **can be an effective means of** weight loss.

Imitation Sentence:

☆ Parenteral vaccination **can be an effective means of** inducing protective mucosal responses.

1) Hypertensive disorders of pregnancy **constitute** one of the leading causes of maternal and perinatal mortality worldwide.

Answer: _____ **constitute** _____

_____

_____

2) Although maternal mortality is much lower in high-income countries than in developing countries, 16% of maternal deaths **can be attributed to** hypertensive disorders.

Answer: _____ **can be**
attributed to _____

3) Preeclampsia with severe features can **result in** acute and long-term
complications for the woman and her newborn.

Answer: _____ **result in** _____

_____

4) Preeclampsia **is** primarily **defined as** gestational hypertension plus proteinuria
(300 mg/24 hours).

Answer: _____ **is defined as** _____

_____

5. **Match the following statements with the corresponding sections in the text.**

Epidemiology: _____   Management: _____

Mechanisms/Pathophysiology: _____   Quality of Life: _____

Diagnosis: _____   Prevention: _____

A. Although hypertension and proteinuria are considered to be the classical
   criteria to diagnose preeclampsia, other criteria are also important.

B. To date, no intervention has been proved unequivocally effective at eliminating
   the risk of preeclampsia.

C. In addition to appropriate management of labor and delivery, the two main
   goals of management of women with preeclampsia during labor and delivery
   are prevention of seizures and control of hypertension.

D. Hypertensive disorders of pregnancy constitute one of the leading causes of
   maternal and perinatal mortality worldwide.

E. Preeclampsia is a disorder of pregnancy associated with new-onset
   hypertension, which occurs most often after 20 weeks of gestation and
   frequently near term.

F. Several mechanisms of disease have been proposed in preeclampsia, including
   the following: chronic uteroplacental ischemia, immune maladaptation, very
   low-density lipoprotein toxicity, genetic imprinting, increased trophoblast
   apoptosis or necrosis, and an exaggerated maternal inflammatory response to
   deported trophoblasts.

6. **Read the introduction in the box and finish the exercises after it.**

> *Division* is one way to sort things out and used to deal with one thing. Its
> purpose is to separate that thing into parts. For example, a pair of glasses
> can be divided into the frame and the lens, and a composition, into
> introduction, body, and conclusion.

1) Single-line the thing to be divided and double-line the parts.

The uterus has four major regions: the fundus, the body, the isthmus, and the cervix. The fundus is the broad curved upper area in which the fallopian tubes connect to the uterus. The body, the main part of the uterus, starts directly below the level of the fallopian tubes and continues downward until the uterine walls and cavity begin to narrow. The isthmus is the lower, narrow neck region. The lowest section, the cervix, extends downward from the isthmus until it opens into the vagina.

2) Reorder the following sentences to make an effective paragraph.

A. Serosa is the smooth outer layer.

B. The uterus has three layers: endometrium, myometrium and serosa.

C. Endometrium is the inner lining.

D. Myometrium is the thick middle muscle layer of the corpus or fundus.

E. It is shed during the period.

F. This expands during pregnancy to hold the growing baby. It contracts during labor to push the baby out.

G. It covers the uterus and makes it easy for the uterus to move in the pelvis as needed.

Answer: __ __ __ __ __ __ __

7. Translate the Chinese paragraph below into English.

先兆子痫指妊娠 24 周左右,在患有高血压、蛋白尿基础上,出现头痛、眼花、恶心、呕吐、上腹不适等症状。先兆子痫患者,尤其是早发型和/或重度先兆子痫患者,晚年发生高血压、缺血性心脏病、卒中、静脉血栓栓塞和相关疾病的风险增加。再次妊娠先兆子痫复发风险大。

8. Read the text and fill in the sheet with proper information.

Reading Prompts	
Items	**Your Answers**
1) Identify the medical terms concerning *preeclampsia* and group them according to your understanding.	
2) Identify the *adjectives* used in "*Diagnosis*" and explain what conditions they describe.	

continued

Reading Prompts	
Items	**Your Answers**
3) *Identify the* **conjunctions** *used in* "**Epidemiology**" *and point out the logical relation each of them indicates.*	
4) *Identify the* **verbs** *used in* **Exercise 3** *and point out the changes of verb tenses.*	
5) *Identify the* **typical sentence patterns**. (**the whole article**)	
6) *Identify the* **topic sentence** *and the supporting sentences in* **paragraph 1 in** "**Mechanisms/Pathophysiology**".	

Title: _____

Although the rise of midwifery as a respected profession varies from country to country, most histories go far back, well before the rise of modern obstetrics. What is often forgotten by modern health systems and policy analysis is that, in most instances, midwifery has not grown out of, or been a specialist branch of nursing, rather it has its origins in social welfare and public health.

Midwifery, as a profession and those who practice midwifery, are less beholden to the teachings and tenants of Florence Nightingale and nursing dogma, than some profess. Although Florence Nightingale did open a school of midwifery, as her own diary shows, she soon closed it and declared, "These midwives were un-trainable!" These midwives she refers to, like the early recruits into midwifery in Africa, were not young women from gentle families, but rather many were married women who themselves had given birth and knew the need for quality care to save the lives of not just the mother, but also the newborn. In many countries in Africa the early history of midwifery owes much to the early missionaries and not armed warfare—which required building a nursing cadre to care for wounded and dying soldiers. Many of the early programs for midwifery were less formal than those for nursing and often seen as being at a lower academic level.

Countries such as Yemen and Sudan, where the majority of the births still take place in the home or community, have for many decades been building their professional midwifery workforce, albeit with limited success to date on community services. In Sudan, since 1926 they have done this by focusing on trying to reach out to women in the community, especially poor communities, to encourage women from these communities to be trained as midwives and then return to their communities to work. Experience from other countries shows that once the community finds these health workers (midwives) acceptable, they are then more willing to seek out their services and to be referred to and in time seek care from maternity facilities that can offer the full range of essential obstetric (and midwifery) care.

Experiences from other countries such as Malaysia and Sri Lanka show that with time, such trust and confidence in the new cadre can be achieved. The focus was on going out to communities and making links and partnerships with the traditional birth attendants (both the trained and non-trained traditional birth attendants) as well as partnerships with physicians. Malaysia initially followed a British model and developed licensing and regulation early in the development of their health system. Midwifery in Malaysia is now a highly specialized training following public health nursing, and midwives are to be found at all levels of the health services, including in rural midwifery-led facilities. Sri Lanka however, despite initial similarities with Malaysia, has not developed their community-based public health midwife. Although some public health midwives have moved from community practice into hospitals where the majority of women now give birth, they are not treated with high regard, but rather must work as auxiliary staff under the supervision of a Registered Nurse who has 6 months additional training in midwifery after nursing program.

It is only in more recent times, across many countries of the world, that for expedience, managers and administrators have grouped midwives and nurses under one professional grouping, and often placing at the head a nurse, rather than a midwife. This subsuming midwifery into nursing has done much to account for both the disappearance of midwifery in some countries, and poor quality of care; as in such cases midwives are no longer able to become expert leaders, academics and researchers to advance the art and science of midwifery. It is only those countries that have been able to hold fast to the identity and autonomy of midwifery, or the newer countries like New Zealand and Canada which have fought hard to create the space and definition of autonomous midwifery practice, which can boast of a strong professional midwife cadre.

The philosophy or midwifery and the real tenants of midwifery practice can be found in empowerment of women, helping pregnant women progress through their pregnancies, give birth to a newborn, and then adjust to the care for this new family member. Because the bringing of new life is as much a social and spiritual activity as it is physical, midwives must have at the center of their practice the elements of social welfare—helping women prepare not only mentally but also physically, such as making savings for the birth, additional food, clothing and other items. However, it is true that midwifery and midwives are not held in high regards in all countries, but often those places where midwives are not given special regards, are also the countries where women's status is low. The narrative of the rise or fall of midwifery is in most cases interlinked with women's lives and status, and too often their poverty and lack of voice.

(Extracted from "The State of the World's Midwifery 2011")

Exercises

1. Read the article and write a possible title for it.

2. Answer the following questions according to the passage.

    1) When did the profession of midwifery appear?

    2) Why did Florence Nightingale close training programs for midwives?

    3) Why did Sudan encourage women from poor communities to be midwives?

    4) What may account for the disappearance of midwifery in some countries?

    5) What do you think about the maternity hotel in China?

UNIT 3 Nephrology

Nephrology deals with the normal working of the kidneys as well as its diseases. The diseases that come under the scope of nephrology include glomerular disorders, urine abnormalities, tubulointerstitial diseases, renal vascular diseases and kidney and bladder stones etc.

Part I Intensive Reading

Kidney Stones

Kidney stones are mineral deposits in the renal calyces and pelvis that are found free or attached to the renal papillae. They contain crystalline and organic components and are formed when the urine becomes supersaturated with a mineral. Calcium oxalate is the main constituent of most stones, many of which form on a foundation of calcium phosphate called Randall's plaques, which are present on the renal papillary surface.

Epidemiology

A recent review of epidemiological data from seven countries revealed incidence rates for kidney stones of 114 – 720 per 100,000 individuals and prevalence rates of 1.7% – 14.8%, and in nearly all countries, the rates seem to be rising.

The propensity to form stones varies according to sex, ethnicity, geography, as well as family and genetic factors. Although historically stones have been 2 to 3 times more common in men than in women, recent data indicate that this disparity is diminishing. The reason for the surge in stone disease in women is not precisely understood, but changes in lifestyle and diet, resulting in increased obesity among women, might have been a known risk factor for stone formation. Racial and ethnic differences in stone prevalence have long been recognized. In the United States, non-Hispanic white individuals have the highest prevalence among racial and ethnic groups, followed by Hispanics and non-Hispanic African Americans. Geographical variation in stone disease typically reflects environmental risk factors, with higher stone prevalence in hot and/or arid climates. After controlling for other factors, ambient temperature and sunlight have been shown to be independently associated with stone prevalence. A positive family history of kidney stones is also an important risk factor; it is present in up to 50% of stone-formers, and first-degree relatives of stone formers are twice as likely to have or develop a stone. Several genes have been implicated or investigated as possible contributors to idiopathic kidney stone risk.

Numerous systemic diseases and factors have been associated with an increased risk of kidney stones. Weight, body mass index and diabetes have been shown in large prospective cohort studies to correlate with the risk of incident kidney stones. Metabolic syndrome has also been linked to risk of kidney stones.

Mechanisms/Pathophysiology

- Calculi types

Kidney stones are solid masses, ranging in size from a grain of sand to a pearl. Depending on their composition, stones are either yellow or brown in color and smooth or jagged in appearance.

The four main types of stones are named after their major constituents. Calcium stones are the most common and occur as CaOx (calcium oxalate) and CaP (calcium phosphate) crystals, alone or in combination. Most kidney stones are partially or completely composed of CaOx, which exists as a monohydrate or dehydrate stones. CaOx stone formation is a multistep process. Hypercalciuria, hyperoxaluria and hypocitraturia are major risk factors. CaP is mainly found as basic CaP (apatite), calcium hydrogen phosphate dihydrate or tricalcium phosphate. Pure CaP stones are rare. Hypercalciuria, hypocitraturia and increased urinary pH are major risk factors for CaP stone formation. Uric acid stones comprise 8%–10% of all kidney stones worldwide. Unlike calcium stone types, overly acidic urine (a pH of <5.5) is recognized as the main abnormality responsible for uric acid nephrolithiasis. In addition to the insolubility of uric acid at low urinary pH and dehydration, conditions that lead to excessive urinary uric acid excretion, known as hyperuricosuria, have also been associated with uric acid stone formation. Struvite stones, also known as "infection stones", represent 7%–8% of all stones worldwide and are typically caused by increased production of ammonia secondary to infection with urease-producing organisms, such as Proteus or Klebsiella. Finally, cystine stones form as result of an autosomal recessive defect in the renal transporter of the amino acid cystine. The lack of cystine reabsorption leads to increased urinary cystine excretion. At normal urinary pH, cystine is insoluble and forms cystine crystals that can aggregate to form recurrent kidney and bladder stones.

• Chemistry of stone formation

Several models of kidney stone formation have been proposed. The two dominating mechanisms for the initiation of stones are commonly described by the terms "free particle" (in which crystals form "Randall's plugs" in the tubule) and "fixed particle" (in which stones grow on so-called Randall's plaques). Although these models encompass all the possible hypothetical models of how stones begin, no single model can rationalize the evidence observed from all patients with stones—many factors probably contribute. Regardless of the model, the chemical processes of nucleation and crystal growth are essential for the initiation and development of all stone types. Stone formation is caused by an abnormal combination of factors that influence the thermodynamic driving force (supersaturation) and the kinetic (rate-controlling) processes involved in the crystallization of the various stone-forming minerals. The principal thermodynamic driving force for both stages is the degree of supersaturation of the fluid within which initiation occurs. Whether this takes place intracellularly or extracellularly, the laws of crystallization chemistry must apply.

Diagnosis

Clinical presentation. Patients with urinary stones generally present with the typical reno-ureteral colic and less frequently with loin pain. Associated manifestations could be gross hematuria, vomiting and sometimes fever. However, patients can also be asymptomatic. A diagnosis of nephrolithiasis is only confirmed when a stone has been passed, has been extracted or destroyed, or has been identified in the urinary tract by imaging studies or surgery.

Medical history. In the diagnosis of the patients, systemic and environmental influences must be carefully identified. Systemic abnormalities include intestinal disease, disorders of calcium homeostasis such as primary hyperparathyroidism, obesity, type II diabetes, recurrent urinary tract infection, bariatric surgery, medullary sponge kidney and various drug treatments.

Laboratory evaluations. Laboratory diagnosis includes stone analysis, imaging studies, blood profiles and a urine metabolic evaluation. Stone analysis plays a valuable role in the diagnosis of kidney stone patients, specifically in infrequently encountered kidney stones such as uric acid, cystine, infection-induced drug-induced and NH4+ urate stones.

Imaging. Several imaging tests are also very important in helping doctors to make the diagnosis of the disease.

□ *Kidney-ureter-bladder (KUB) X-ray.* Urinary calculi that are rich in calcium are radio-opaque. Stones containing calcium phosphate are usually the most radio-opaque with a density similar to bone; calcium oxalate stones are very opaque and cannot usually be distinguished from calcium phosphate stones. Magnesium ammonium phosphate (struvite) stones are less radio-opaque; radiolucent stones include pure cystine or uric acid, xanthine, dihydroxyadenine, indinavir, triamterene and matrix.

□ *Ultrasound.* Ultrasound scanning is a useful and safer screening method when following patients with a history of recurrent stones.

□ *Intravenous urogram (IVU).* The administration of intravenous contrast media is still a useful investigation in diagnosing an obstructing urinary tract stone as there will be a delay in the appearance of contrast in the renal parenchyma and collecting system.

□ *Computed tomography of kidneys, ureters and bladder(CT-KUB).* An un-enhanced CT scan is now the gold standard investigation in the diagnosis of urinary tract stones in an emergency. The CT-KUB is reported to have a sensitivity of 97% and a specificity of 96%. The scans can be done rapidly and do not require contrast, and they are cost-effective when compared with an IVU.

Management

- Surgical management

Over the past 30 years, the management of pediatric and adult patients with symptomatic kidney stones has evolved from open surgical lithotomy to minimally invasive endourological treatments leading to a reduction in patient morbidity, improved stone-free rates and better quality of life. The three most common treatment modalities for kidney stones are listed below.

Shockwave lithotripsy (SWL). SWL involves the non-invasive delivery of high-energy acoustic waves that fragment a kidney stone. When these shockwaves approach and pass through the calculus, energy is released resulting in internal structure disruption and stone fragmentation. It remains the most commonly performed endourological kidney stone procedure worldwide.

Ureteroscopic fragmentation and retrieval. Ureteroscopy consists of retrograde passage of an endoscope from the urethra proximally towards the affected ureter and kidney, enabling access to the stone as well as delivery of other instruments, such as guidewires, balloon dilators, laser fibers and baskets. Ureteroscopy is favored over SWL in the setting of multiple or radiolucent stones, hydronephrosis, obesity or high-density stones.

Percutaneous nephrolithotomy (PCNL). PCNL involves the direct passage of an endoscope percutaneously through skin, muscle and perirenal fat, and into the kidney and is generally performed for stones >2 cm in size.

- Medical management

Treatment of renal colic and medical expulsive therapy. Treatment of the pain (renal colic) associated with kidney stones is based on the use of nonsteroidal anti-inflammatory drugs as a first choice in the absence of contraindication and, in case of failure in relieving pain, opioids. Intravenous paracetamol also seems to be as effective as morphine. Alpha adrenergic receptor antagonists and calcium channel blockers have been demonstrated to be an effective medical expulsive therapy, believed to be due to their ability to dilate the distal ureter and increase the probability of spontaneous stone passage.

Oral and percutaneous dissolution therapy of stones. Oral dissolution of existing stones is generally effective only with uric acid stones. Two-thirds of these stones can be at least partially dissolved by following the same rules suggested for their prevention: modulating the pH of urine to 7.0, increasing urinary volume, and decreasing uricosuria with allopurinol. A few observations also suggest that cystine stones might be amenable to oral chemolysis with 6-mercaptopropionyl glycine, high urine output and alkalization. Finally, the use of percutaneous solutions, such as 10% hemiacidrin or Suby's solution, to turn insoluble kidney stones into more-water-soluble forms was popularized in the 1960s but is rarely used today. Although somewhat effective for infection, uric acid, cystine and brushite stones, percutaneous dissolution of kidney stones is labor intensive and considerably less effective than contemporary minimally invasive removal techniques.

Quality of Life

As indicated earlier, the prevalence of urolithiasis and nephrolithiasis has increased over the past decades and affects approximately 9% of the adult population. Although many kidney stones remain asymptomatic for long periods, the incidence of stone episodes, such as pain, infection or obstruction, has increased. Furthermore, following an initial stone event, >50% of patients experience a recurrent stone in the following 5 years. Thus, for these patients, treatment (both medical and surgical) and implementation of lifestyle modifications can significantly affect the patient's QoL.

Prevention

Effective kidney stone prevention depends upon addressing the cause of stone formation. Proper management of diet and the use of medications is required. Patients should be instructed to increase their water intake in order to maintain a urine output of at least 2 liter per day. Restriction of animal proteins is also encouraged since animal proteins provide an increased acid load because of its high content of sulfur-containing amino acid. People who form calcium stones used to be told to avoid dairy products and other foods with high calcium content. They should not be advised to restrict calcium intake unless it has been known that they have an excessive use of calcium.

(Extracted from *Nature*)

Vocabulary

calyces	['keɪlɪsiːz]	*n.*	肾盏
pelvis	['pelvɪs]	*n.*	骨盆；肾盂
papillae	[pə'pɪli]	*n.*	乳突
supersaturated	[suːpər'sætʃəreɪtɪd]	*adj.*	过饱和的
propensity	[prə'pensəti]	*n.*	倾向；习性
arid	['ærɪd]	*adj.*	干燥的；不毛的
ambient	['æmbɪənt]	*adj.*	周围的；氛围的
idiopathic	[ˌɪdɪə'pæθɪk]	*adj.*	先天的；特发的
jagged	['dʒægɪd]	*adj.*	参差不齐的
oxalate	['ɒksəˌleɪt]	*n.*	草酸盐
monohydrate	[ˌmɒnəʊ'haɪdreɪt]	*n.*	一水合物
hypercalciuria	[ˌhaɪpəˌkælsɪ'juːərɪə]	*n.*	高钙尿
hyperoxaluria	[haɪprɒk'sælʊərɪə]	*n.*	高草酸尿症
apatite	['æpətaɪt]	*n.*	磷灰石
dihydrate	[daɪ'haɪdreɪt]	*n.*	二水合物
tricalcium	[traɪ'kælsɪəm]	*n.*	三钙
acidic	[ə'sɪdɪk]	*adj.*	酸的；酸性的
nephrolithiasis	[nefrəʊlɪ'θaɪəsɪs]	*n.*	肾石病
hyperuricosuria	[haɪprʊərɪ'kəʊsjʊːrɪə]	*n.*	高尿酸尿

struvite	['struːvaɪt]	n. 鸟粪石
ammonia	[ə'məʊnɪə]	n. 氨
urease	['jʊərɪeɪs]	n. 脲酶；尿素酶
colic	['kɒlɪk]	n. 腹绞痛
hyperparathyroidism	[haɪpəpærə'θaɪrɒɪdɪzəm]	n. 甲状旁腺功能亢进
bariatric	[ˌbærɪ'ætrɪk]	adj. 肥胖病治疗学的
radio-opaque	['reɪdiːəʊəʊp'eɪk]	adj. 射线透不过的
radiolucent	['reɪdɪəʊ'luːsnt]	adj. 射线可透过的
urogram	[ərəg'ræm]	n. 尿路造影照片
tomography	[tə'mɒɡrəfi]	n. X线断层摄影术
lithotomy	[lɪ'θɒtəmɪ]	n. 切石术
lithotripsy	['lɪθəʊˌtrɪpsi]	n. 碎石术
ureteroscopy	[jʊəriːtə'rɒskəpɪ]	n. 输尿管镜检查术
hydronephrosis	[ˌhaɪdrəʊnɪ'frəʊsɪs]	n. 肾盂积水
opioid	[əʊ'piːəʊɪd]	n. 类鸦片
paracetamol	[ˌpærə'siːtəmɒl]	n. 扑热息痛
expulsive	[ɪk'spʌlsɪv]	adj. 逐出的
uricosuria	[jʊːrɪ'kəʊsjuːrɪə]	n. 尿酸尿
allopurinol	[æləʊ'pjʊərɪnɒl]	n. 别嘌呤醇
chemolysis	[kɪ'mɒləsɪs]	n. 化学溶蚀
mercaptopropionyl	[məːkæptɒprəʊpa'ɪɒnɪl]	n. 巯丙酰
glycine	['glaɪsiːn]	n. 甘氨酸；氨基乙酸
alkalization	[ælkəlaɪ'zeɪʃən]	n. 碱性化
hemiacidrin	[hiːmiːæ'sɪdrɪn]	n. 溶肾石酸素
sulfur	['sʌlfə(r)]	n. 硫（磺）

Exercises

1. **Read the text and explain the following medical phrases.**

   1) Risk factors for kidney stones
   2) Major risk factors for CaP stone
   3) Types of kidney stones
   4) Treating modalities for kidney stones
   5) Mechanisms for the initiation of kidney stones

2. **Answer the following questions according to the text.**

   1) How do patients with kidney stones present?
   2) What imaging tests can be used to diagnose kidney stones?

3) Why is the percutaneous solution seldom used today?

4) Do you know how to prevent kidney stones?

3. Fill in the blanks with the proper forms of the given words.

diarrhea	perspiration	solute	fluid	intake
crystal	urine	surgery	calculus	output

Thorough and detailed investigation identifies an underlying cause for 1)_____ formation in over 90% of cases. Low 2)_____ volume is the most important factor contributing to calculus formation and growth. There is a lower limit to the amount of urinary 3)_____ that has to be excreted each day, so a low urine volume inevitably causes concentrated urine. Some substances will be present in concentrations at the upper limit of their solubility, leading to precipitation of 4)_____, which aggregate into calculi. A low urine volume results from an oral fluid intake insufficient to maintain a normal 24-hour urine 5)_____ of, ideally, at least 1.5 liters in a temperate climate. A low oral fluid 6)_____ is an occasional cause of low urine volume, especially in old age or in occupational or other circumstances which limit the facility to drink frequently. Much more common is the situation where extra-urinary 7)_____ loss is excessive. This can occur in situations of chronic 8)_____ or after some forms of bowel 9)_____ but excessive fluid loss by sweating is by far the most important cause. Oral fluid intake needs to exceed 10)_____ losses by at least 2 liters to maintain satisfactory urine volume.

4. Study the bold-faced words in each of the following sentences and imitate the particular way of writing.

Mentor Sentence:

☆ In morbidly obese patients, bariatric surgery **can be an effective means of** weight loss.

Imitation Sentence:

☆ Parenteral vaccination **can be an effective means of** inducing protective mucosal responses.

1) A recent review of epidemiological data from seven countries **revealed** incidence rates **for** kidney stones **of** 114 – 720 per 100,000 individuals and prevalence rates of 1.7%–14.8%.

Answer: _____ **revealed** _____ **for**

_____ **of** _____

_____

2) Kidney stones are solid masses, **ranging in size from** a grain of sand **to** a pearl.

Answer: _____ **ranging in size from** __

_____ **to** _____

3) **Patients with** urinary stones generally **present with** the typical reno-ureteral colic **and less frequently with** loin pain

Answer: **Patients with** _____ **present with** _____

_____ **and less frequently with** _____

4) **Over** the past 30 years, **the management of** pediatric and adult patients with symptomatic kidney stones **has evolved from** open surgical lithotomy **to** minimally invasive endourological approaches.

Answer: **Over** _____, **the management of** _____ **has**

evolved from _____ **to** _____

_____

5. **Match the following statements with the corresponding sections in the text.**

Epidemiology: _____ Quality of Life: _____

Management: _____ Diagnosis: _____

Mechanisms/Pathophysiology: _____ Prevention: _____

A. Management of symptomatic kidney stones has evolved from open surgical lithotomy to minimally invasive endourological treatments leading to a reduction in patient morbidity, improved stone-free rates and better quality of life.

B. The prevalence of stones has been consistently increasing over the past 50 years and further increases are expected owing to changing lifestyle, dietary habits and global warming.

C. Obesity, diabetes, hypertension, and metabolic syndrome are considered risk factors for stone formation.

D. Prevention of recurrence requires behavioral and nutritional interventions, as well as pharmacological treatments that are specific for the type of stone.

E. There is a great need for recurrence prevention that requires a better understanding of the mechanisms involved in stone formation to facilitate the development of more-effective drugs.

F. Stones that develop in the urinary tract (known as nephrolithiasis or urolithiasis) form when the urine becomes excessively supersaturated with respect to a mineral, leading to crystal formation, growth, aggregation and retention within the kidneys.

G. Renal calculi are renowned for their tendency to recur, even after apparently satisfactory treatment.

H. Multiple imaging modalities are available, but widespread clinical use is currently limited to CT, ultrasonography, and kidney ureter bladder (KUB) plain film radiography.

6. Read the introduction in the box and finish the exercises after it.

> *Classification is another way of sorting things out. Division is used to deal with one thing. Classification, on the other hand, is used to organize things which share certain qualities. Its purpose is to group these things systematically. The same group of things can be classified into categories according to one principle. Classification deals with the parts and division, the whole.*

1) Single-line the item to be classified, double-line the principle to classify and circle the classified categories.

    The four main types of stones are named after their major constituents. Calcium stones are the most common and occur as CaOx (calcium oxalate) and CaP (calcium phosphate) crystals, alone or in combination. Uric acid stones comprise 8%–10% of all kidney stones worldwide. Unlike calcium stone types, overly acidic urine (a pH of < 5.5) is recognized as the main abnormality responsible for uric acid nephrolithiasis. Struvite stones, also known as "infection stones", represent 7%–8% of all stones worldwide and are typically caused by increased production of ammonia secondary to infection with urease-producing organisms, such as Proteus or Klebsiella. Finally, cystine stones form as result of an autosomal recessive defect in the renal transporter of the amino acid cystine. The lack of cystine reabsorption leads to increased urinary cystine excretion.

2) Reorder the following sentences to make an effective paragraph.

A. Depending on the results of the stone analysis, a patient may be instructed to make dietary changes, such as lowering salt and protein, avoiding foods with high oxalate content, and eating foods less in calcium.

B. Patients can avoid future kidney stones by preventing the materials that can form stones from concentrating in the urine.

C. Kidney stones from calcium salts can be prevented by using diuretics such as hydrochlorothiazide or chlorthalidone, along with potassium citrate to increase urine pH.

D. Prevention of uric acid stones may require the use of allopurinol and potassium citrate.

E. Maintaining good hydration by drinking plenty of water each day is a key to prevention.

F. Struvite stones can be prevented by small doses of antibiotic taken daily.

Answer： __ __ __ __ __ __

7. Translate the Chinese paragraph below into English.

尿石病是泌尿系统的常见疾病,可见于肾、膀胱、输尿管和尿道的任何部位,但以肾与输尿管结石为常见。结石形成病因十分复杂,与全身代谢、泌尿系统局部感染和饮食因素有密切关系,明确的病因有甲亢、肾小管酸中毒、海绵肾、痛风、异物、长期卧床、梗阻及感染等。

8. Read the text and fill in the sheet with proper information.

Reading Prompts	
Items	**Your Answers**
1) *Identify the medical terms concerning **kidney stones** and group them according to your understanding.*	
2) *Identify the **adjectives** used in **"Clinical presentation"** and explain what conditions they describe.*	
3) *Identify the **conjunctions** used in **"Quality of Life"** and point out the logical relation each of them indicates.*	
4) *Identify the **verbs** used in **"Epidemiology"** and point out the changes of verb tenses. (**Epidemiology**)*	
5) *Identify the **typical sentence patterns**. (**the whole article**)*	
6) *Identify the **topic sentence** and the **supporting sentences** in **"Prevention"**.*	

Part II   Extensive Reading

Title: _____

The first scientific description of treatment procedures for kidney failure procedures dates back to the 19th century and came from the Scottish chemist Thomas Graham, who became known as the "Father of Dialysis".

Today hemodialysis describes an extracorporeal procedure, or procedure outside the body, for filtering uremic substances from the blood of patients suffering from kidney disease.

The Early Days of Dialysis

The first historical description of this type of procedure was published in 1913. Abel, Rowntree, and Turner "dialyzed" anesthetized animals by directing their blood outside the body and through tubes of semipermeable membranes made from collodion.

A German doctor by the name of Georg Haas performed the first dialysis treatments involving humans. It is believed that Haas dialyzed the first patient with kidney failure at the University of Giessen in the summer of 1924. By 1928, Haas had dialyzed an additional six patients, none of whom survived, likely because of the critical condition of the patients and the insufficient effectiveness of the dialysis treatment.

The First Successful Dialysis Treatment

In the fall of 1945, Willem Kolff of the Netherlands, made the breakthrough that had stubbornly eluded Haas. Kolff used a rotating drum kidney he had developed to perform a week-long dialysis treatment on a 67-year-old patient who had been admitted to hospital with acute kidney failure. The patient was subsequently discharged with normal kidney function. This patient proved that the concept developed by Abel and Haas could be put into practice and thus represented the first major breakthrough in the treatment of patients with kidney disease.

The Rotating Drum Kidney

Examples of the Kolff rotating drum kidney crossed the Atlantic and arrived at the Peter Brent Brigham Hospital in Boston, where they underwent a significant technical improvement. The modified machines became known as the Kolff-Brigham artificial kidney, and between 1954 and 1962 were shipped from Boston to 22 hospitals worldwide. The Kolff-Brigham kidney had previously passed its practical test under extreme conditions during the Korean War. Dialysis treatment succeeded in improving the average survival rate of soldiers suffering from post-traumatic kidney failure.

Dialysis and Ultrafiltration

One of the most important functions of the natural kidney, in addition to the filtering of uremic toxins, is the removal of excess water. When the kidneys fail, this function must be taken over by the artificial kidney, which is also known as a dialyzer. The procedure by which plasma water from the patient is squeezed through the dialyzer membrane using pressure is termed ultrafiltration. In 1947, Swede Nils Alwall published a scientific work describing a modified dialyzer that could perform the necessary combination of dialysis and ultrafiltration better than the original Kolff kidney. The cellophane membranes used in this dialyzer could withstand higher pressure because of their positioning between two protective metal grates.

Further Developments

By proving that uremic patients could be successfully treated using the artificial kidney, Kolff sparked a flurry of activity around the world to develop improved and more effective dialyzers. The "Parallel Plate Dialyzer" evolved as the most significant development of this period. Rather than pumping the blood through membranous tubes, this dialyzer directed the flow of dialysis solution and blood through alternating layers of membranous material.

Just as the technology of dialyzers continued to develop, so too did the scientific principles regarding the transport of substances across membranes, and these principles were applied specifically to dialysis. This work enabled scientists to develop a quantitative description of the dialysis process and allowed the development of dialyzers with clearly defined characteristics.

Vascular Access and Chronic Dialysis

Belding Scribner made a breakthrough in this field in 1960 in the United States with the development of what would later become known as the "Scribner shunt". This new method provided a relatively simple means of accessing a patient's circulatory system that could be used over a period of several months, meaning that patients with chronic kidney disease could, for the first time, be treated with dialysis.

Still, the most decisive breakthrough in the field of vascular access came in 1966 from Michael Brescia and James Cimino. Their work remains fundamentally important to dialysis today. The arteriovenous (AV) fistula remains the access of choice for dialysis patients and some AV fistula implanted more than 30 years ago are still in use today.

Modern Hemodialysis

After the early successes in Seattle, hemodialysis established itself as the treatment of choice worldwide for chronic and acute kidney failure. Membranes, dialyzers and dialysis machines were continuously improved and manufactured industrially in ever increasing numbers. A major step forward was the development of the first hollow fiber dialyzer in 1964. This procedure allowed for the production of dialyzers with a surface area large enough to fulfill the demands of efficient dialysis treatment. Over the years that followed, thanks to the development of appropriate industrial manufacturing technologies, it became possible to produce large numbers of disposable dialyzers at a reasonable price. Today, dialyzers are made from entirely synthetic polysulfone, a plastic that exhibits exceptionally good filtering efficiency and tolerability for patients.

State-of-the-art dialysis machines also monitor patients to ensure critical conditions can be detected at an early stage and treated. They feature efficient monitoring and data management systems and have become more user-friendly over recent years. A growing number of the latest generation of dialysis machines also utilize computer-controlled machines, online technologies, networking and special software.

(Extracted from https://www.fresenius.com/history-of-dialysis)

Exercises

1. **Read the article and write a possible title for it.**

2. **Answer the following questions according to the passage.**

　　1) Who is the "Father of Dialysis"?

　　2) How did the Kolff-Brigham kidney pass its practical test?

　　3) Why is Michael Brescia and James Cimino's work still important today?

　　4) What is the advantage of the first hollow-fiber dialyzer?

　　5) Do you agree that being a good listener is critical to being a good doctor? Why, or why not?

UNIT 4 Infectious Diseases

Infectious diseases are disorders caused by organisms—including bacteria, viruses, fungi and parasites. In 2006, most frequently reported infectious diseases in China were tuberculosis, hepatitis B, dysentery, syphilis, and gonorrhea, accounting for 3,963,663 of 4,608,910 (86%) reported cases of the 27 notifiable infectious diseases.

Part I   Intensive Reading

Tuberculosis

Tuberculosis (TB) is a contagious disease that is transmitted from person to person through coughing and breathing in airborne droplets that contain bacteria. TB primarily affects the lungs but can affect any part of the body. As one of the most common infections in the world, TB remains a major problem in many countries and among vulnerable populations.

Epidemiology

Tuberculosis is the leading cause of death from a curable infectious disease. According to surveys, there were an estimated 8.9 million new cases of tuberculosis in 2004. About 3.9 million cases were sputum-smear positive, the most infectious form of the disease. The WHO African region has the highest estimated incidence rate (356 per 100,000 population per year), but the majority of patients with tuberculosis live in the most populous countries of Asia: Bangladesh, India, Indonesia, Pakistan etc. together account for half (48%) the new cases that arise every year. About 80% of individuals newly diagnosed with the disease every year live in the 22 most populous countries.

Much of the increase in global tuberculosis incidence seen since 1980 is attributable to the spread of HIV in Africa. In African populations with high rates of HIV infection, a relatively high proportion of patients with tuberculosis are women aged 15 to 24 years. The rise in the number of tuberculosis cases is slowing in Africa, almost certainly because HIV infection rates are beginning to stabilize or fall. HIV has probably had a smaller effects on tuberculosis prevalence than on incidence because the virus significantly reduces the life expectancy of patients with tuberculosis.

Mechanisms/Pathophysiology

Inhalation of Mycobacterium tuberculosis leads to one of four possible outcomes:

- □ *immediate clearance of the organism*
- □ *latent infection*
- □ *the onset of active disease (primary disease)*
- □ *active disease many years later (reactivation disease)*

Among individuals with latent infection, and no underlying medical problems, reactivation disease occurs in 5 to 10 percent of cases. The risk of reactivation is markedly increased in patients with HIV. These outcomes are determined by the interplay of factors attributable to both the organism and the host. Among the approximately 10% of infected individuals who develop active disease, about half will develop rapidly progressive or primary disease.

The tubercle bacilli establish infection in the lungs after they are carried in droplets small enough (5 – 10 microns) to reach the alveolar spaces. If the defense system of the host fails to eliminate the infection, the bacilli proliferate inside alveolar macrophages and eventually kill the cells. The infected macrophages produce cytokines and chemokines that attract other phagocytic cells, including monocytes, other alveolar macrophages and neutrophils, which eventually form a nodular granulomatous structure called the tubercle. If the bacterial replication is not controlled, the tubercle enlarges, and the bacilli enter local draining lymph nodes. This leads to lymphadenopathy, a characteristic clinical manifestation of primary tuberculosis. The lesion produced by the expansion of the tubercle into the lung parenchyma and lymph node involvement is called the Ghon complex. Bacteremia may accompany initial infection.

The bacilli continue to proliferate until an effective cell-mediated immune (CMI) response develops, usually two to six weeks after infection. Failure by the host to mount an effective CMI response and tissue repair leads to progressive destruction of the lung. Tumor necrosis factor (TNF)-alpha, reactive oxygen and nitrogen intermediates and the contents of cytotoxic cells may all contribute to the development of caseating necrosis that characterizes a tuberculous lesion.

Unchecked bacterial growth may lead to hematogenous spread of bacilli to produce disseminated TB. Disseminated disease with lesions resembling millet seeds is termed miliary TB including lymph node TB, skeletal (bone and joint) TB, meningitis, gastrointestinal TB, abdominal TB and TB of the kidneys.

Bacilli can also spread by erosion of the caseating lesions into the lung airways and the host becomes infectious to others. In the absence of treatment, death ensues in 80% of cases. The remaining patients develop chronic disease or recover. Chronic disease is characterized by repeated episodes of healing by fibrotic changes around the lesions and tissue breakdown. Complete spontaneous eradication of the bacilli is rare.

Reactivation TB results from proliferation of a previously dormant bacterium seeded at the time of the primary infection. Among individuals with latent infection and no underlying medical problems, reactivation disease occurs in 5%-10%. Immunosuppression is associated with reactivation TB, although it is not clear what specific host factors maintain the infection in a latent state and what triggers the latent infection to become overt. The disease process in reactivation TB tends to be localized (in contrast to primary disease): there is little regional lymph node involvement and less caseation. The lesion typically occurs at the lung apices and disseminated disease is unusual unless the host is severely immunosuppressed. It is generally believed that successfully contained latent TB confers protection against subsequent TB exposure.

Diagnosis

Clinical presentation. TB symptoms are usually gradual in onset and duration varying from weeks to months, although more acute onset can occur in young children or immunocompromised individuals. The typical triad of fever, night sweats and weight loss are present in roughly 75%, 45% and 55% of patients respectively, while a persistent non-remitting cough is the most frequently reported symptom (95%).

Types of TB. There are two forms of the disease:
□ *latent TB without symptoms*
□ *active TB with typical symptoms of cough, phlegm, chest pain, weakness, weight loss, fever, chills and sweating at night*

Diagnosis of Tuberculosis. A diagnosis of tuberculosis can sometimes be quite a difficult and laborious process. This is because tuberculosis can sometimes be active, but in some individuals, it can be latent.

The first step in making a diagnosis of TB is a **clinical history**. The physician treating the patient must be able to determine whether the symptoms point towards tuberculosis or not. This can sometimes be quite difficult given the symptoms are rather vague at times.

Once the clinical suspicion of tuberculosis exists, further investigations are required to confirm the diagnosis. In those individuals who have pulmonary tuberculosis, a **sputum examination** may be done to look for the bacteria. Those individuals who have latent tuberculosis may not express the bacteria in the sputum. So usually, the following tests are helpful to confirm the disease.

- Mantoux test

Here, an extract made from dead mycobacterium is injected right under the surface of the skin. This injection leads to an allergic response characterized by swelling, redness and firmness of the injected area. The presence of all three of these in a significant manner is a positive test. If there is no firmness or redness, the test is negative.

- Chest X-ray

A chest X-ray is a very useful test in the diagnosis of pulmonary tuberculosis. A lot of times however, the chest X-ray can be normal. In those who have active tuberculosis, there can be present patches in the upper part of the lung which are rather diagnostic of the problem. In miliary tuberculosis, the infection can be a lot more widespread and appears like multiple patches all through the lung fields.

- Blood tests

Sometimes, the blood tests performed to diagnose tuberculosis can be negative for the presence of any infection.

- Ultrasound scan of the abdomen

An ultrasound scan is a useful way to determine if there is any infection or abnormality within the abdomen.

- Urine test

In tuberculosis that affects the bladder, the urine will show the presence of pus cells. However, when a urine culture test is performed, there will be no bacteria present. This is called sterile pyuria and is characteristic of tuberculosis of the bladder.

- CT scan of the brain

When tuberculosis affects the brain, a CT scan can help determine the extent to which it is affected. Sometimes, an MRI scan may be required.

Management

Initiating treatment without delay is the only way TB can be cured. Specialized treatment is based on whether TB is an active disease or only an infection. Someone who has been infected but does not have the disease may require preventive therapy only. This preventive therapy is designed to kill the germs that have the potential to cause harm. Preventive therapy is usually a prescription for a daily dose of isoniazid, which is an inexpensive tuberculosis medication. This preventive therapy lasts for nine months, with periodic checkups to ensure the medication being taken correctly.

Active TB cases require treatment with effective drugs, such as: isoniazid, rifampin, pyrazinamide and ethambutol. The treatment regimen entails an initial two-month treatment phase followed by a continuation phase. The continuation phase is suggested to last four months for the majority of patients but can be extended to seven to nine months. All TB medications should be taken together instead of divided doses. Taking the medications correctly is very important due to the fact that if taken incorrectly the patient can become sick and the TB will be more difficult to cure as it becomes drug resistant. Multi drug-resistant TB (MDR TB) is extremely dangerous as the bacteria become resistant to the medication used to treat TB, which makes the treatment ineffective. MDR TB is generally due to the organism becoming resistant to the isoniazid or rifampin, which are the two most important anti-TB medications. Directly observed therapy (DOT) is utilized to ensure that the patients adhere to the therapy set up for them. DOT is an adherence-enhancing strategy in which a designated person watches the patient swallow each dose of medication. This is a recommended practice for all patients when unable to determine who will be compliant and who will not.

Quality of Life

In general, QoL of TB patients is poorer as compared to healthy individuals across most domains, with physical functioning domain affected more severely than others. Although most patients report normal or near-normal QoL after successful TB treatment, a small proportion can still show residual impairment of psychological wellbeing and social functioning. Thus, TB control programs need to look beyond clinical and microbiological aspects, and try to include socio-cultural and psychological dimensions that impact the disease and its treatment. TB patients receiving adequate social support from family, friends and community are likely to have better QoL.

Prevention

There are five ways to prevent tuberculosis.

1. Vaccination: all new born and infants should be given the Bacillus Calmette-Guérin (BCG) vaccine to protect them against TB.

2. Keep immunity high: a healthy lifestyle is important to prevent TB.

3. Maintain good hygiene: simple hygienic practices like covering the mouth while coughing, refraining from spitting in public places are still ignored by people, including those infected with TB.

4. Go to specialist: if you notice any of the symptoms of TB, visit a doctor immediately.

5. Adherence to medication: TB patients do play an important role in preventing the spread of the disease. It is very important for them to complete the prescribed course of treatment due to the strong transmission of the disease.

(Extracted from https://www. researchgate. net)

Vocabulary

mycobacterium	[ˌmaɪkəʊbækˈtɪərɪəm]	n. 分枝杆菌
alveolar	[ælˈviːələ(r)]	adj. 肺泡的;齿槽的
cytokine	[ˈsaɪtəʊˌkaɪn]	n. 细胞因子
neutrophil	[ˈnjʊːtrəˌfɪl]	n. 嗜中性粒细胞
necrosis	[neˈkrəʊsɪs]	n. 坏死;坏疽
hematogenous	[ˌheməˈtɒdʒənəs]	adj. 造血的
eradication	[ɪˌrædɪˈkeɪʃn]	n. 消灭,扑灭;根除
miliary	[mɪlɪˌerɪ]	adj. 粟粒状的;粟粒大的
sterile	[ˈsteraɪl]	adj. 不育的;无菌的
regimen	[ˈredʒɪmən]	n. 养生法;生活规则
smear	[smɪə(r)]	n. 涂片
nodular	[ˈnɒdjʊlə(r)]	adj. 结节状的
granulomatous	[ˌgrænjʊˈləʊmətəs]	adj. 肉芽肿的
tubercle	[ˈtjʊːbəkl]	n. 结节;小瘤
lymphadenopathy	[lɪmˌfædɪˈnɒpəθɪ]	n. 淋巴结病
bacilli	[bəˈsɪlaɪ]	n. 杆菌(bacillus 的复数)
meningitis	[ˌmenɪnˈdʒaɪtɪs]	n. 脑膜炎
apices	[ˈeɪpɪsiːz]	n. 顶端(apex 的复数)
caseation	[ˌkeɪsɪˈeɪʃ(ə)n]	n. 干酪样变;干酪化

| pyuria | [paɪˈjʊərɪə] | n. 脓尿 |
| isoniazid | [ˌaɪsəʊˈnaɪəzɪd] | n. 异烟肼（抗结核药） |

Exercises

1. Read the text and explain the following medical phrases.

1) Transmission of tuberculosis

2) Pathological features of tuberculosis

3) Tools used to diagnose tuberculosis

4) Clinical presentations of tuberculosis

5) Guideline to manage active tuberculosis

2. Answer the following questions according to the text.

1) What are the reasons for the slowing of tuberculosis in Africa?

2) What could lead to lymphadenopathy of primary tuberculosis?

3) Why is it difficult to diagnose tuberculosis?

4) Why is prevention important in TB management?

3. Fill in the blanks with the proper forms of the given words.

| smear | mycobacteria | tuberculosis | sensitive | amplify |
| clinic | control | identify | detect | serology |

1) _____ still remains a major health problem in many developing countries, despite continuous long-standing vaccination and surveillance programs, and worldwide availability of effective anti-tuberculosis drugs. Early 2)_____ is of major importance in the control of tuberculosis. Therefore, a fast and reliable diagnosis of tuberculosis would greatly improve the 3)_____ of tuberculosis. Conventional methods for the diagnosis of tuberculosis, such as the 4)_____ and culture methods have some limitations, particularly the low specificity and 5)_____ as well as the time-consuming nature. Now these limitations have been overcome in some novel and rapid detection methods. Various gene 6)_____ techniques have demonstrated their usefulness in the identification of 7)_____ and its various species. The rapid detection of M. tuberculosis by probes, PCR or other molecular techniques and some newest 8)_____ assays offer good opportunities to improve the diagnosis and therapy of tuberculosis. However, despite the availability of diagnostic tools for laboratory 9)_____ of tuberculosis at high sensitivity and specificity, the "simple and economical" aspect of those new methods is still a matter of

consideration. The question is whether they can be used in simple 10)_____ settings and whether they are economically affordable for developing countries, in most of which tuberculosis is still rampant.

4. **Study the bold-faced words in each of the following sentences and imitate the particular way of writing.**

   Mentor Sentence:

   ☆ In morbidly obese patients, bariatric surgery **can be an effective means of** weight loss.

   Imitation Sentence:

   ☆ Parenteral vaccination **can be an effective means of** inducing protective mucosal responses.

   1) **As** one of the most common infections in the world, TB **remains a major problem in** many countries and among vulnerable populations.

   Answer: **As** _____ , _____ **remain/s a major problem in** _____

   2) Much of the increase in global tuberculosis incidence seen since 1980 **is attributable to** the spread of HIV in Africa.

   Answer: _____ **is/are attributable to** _____
   _____

   3) **The risk of reactivation is markedly increased** in patients with HIV.

   Answer: _____ **is/are markedly increased in** _____
   _____

   4) An ultrasound scan **is a useful way to determine** if there is any infection or abnormality within the abdomen.

   Answer: _____ **is a useful way to determine** _____
   _____

5. **Match the following statements with the corresponding sections in the text.**

   Epidemiology:_____   Management:_____
   Mechanisms/Pathophysiology: _____   Quality of Life:_____
   Diagnosis:_____   Prevention:_____

   A. Good drugs such as isoniazid, rifampin, pyrazinamide and ethambutol are essential to the treatment of active tuberculosis patients.

   B. HIV spread in Africa has led to great increase in global tuberculosis incidence since 1980.

   C. About half of 10% of infected individuals with active disease will develop rapidly progressive or primary disease.

   D. The individuals with pulmonary tuberculosis usually undergo a sputum examination to look for the bacteria.

E. Besides clinical and microbiological aspects, TB control projects need to include socio-cultural and psychological dimensions as part of evaluation and monitoring tools of life quality.

F. Some people infected with TB still pay no attention to simple hygienic practices like covering the mouth while coughing, and refraining from spitting in public places.

G. Isoniazid is an inexpensive tuberculosis medication, so people usually take it daily for preventive therapy.

H. TB symptoms are usually gradual in onset and duration varying from weeks to months, although more acute onset can occur in young children or immunocompromised individuals.

I. The tubercle gets larger and the bacilli go into local draining lymph nodes when the replication of bacteria is uncontrolled.

6. Read the introduction in the box and finish the exercises after it.

> *In composition, **cause and effects** is a method of paragraph development in which a writer analyzes the reasons for—and/or the consequences of—an action, event or a decision. The cause-and-effect pattern may be used to identify one or more causes followed by one or more effects or results. A cause states why something happens. An effects states a result or outcome. At times, **a single cause leads to several effects**. Other times, **several causes contribute to a single effect**. **A causal chain** is a sequence of events in which any one event in the chain causes the next one, leading up to a final effect.*

1) Circle the single cause and underline the effects.

Tuberculosis (TB) is a dangerous and highly contagious bacterial disease caused by mycobacterium tuberculosis. It primarily affects the lungs, but if left untreated, it might spread to different parts of the body. Back pain and stiffness are common complications of tuberculosis. Arthritis that results from tuberculosis (tuberculous arthritis) usually affects the hips and knees. Liver and kidneys help filter waste and impurities from your bloodstream and tuberculosis in these organs can impair their functions.

2) Reorder the following sentences to make an effective paragraph.

A. It is usually associated with concomitant pulmonary TB, and it is thus a highly bacilliferous and contagious form of the disease.

B. Laryngeal tuberculosis usually entails the development of masses, ulcers, or nodules in the larynx and vocal cords, which are usually mistaken as laryngeal neoplasms.

C. The most common clinical manifestation is dysphonia，but it can also produce coughing，stridor and hemoptysis.

Answer：__　__　__

7．Translate the Chinese paragraph below into English.

  肺结核是一种传染性疾病，通过咳嗽和吸入空气中含有细菌的飞沫在人与人之间传播。结核病主要影响肺部，但也可影响身体的任何部位。肺结核有两种形式，即无症状的潜伏性肺结核和活动性肺结核，后者的典型症状为咳嗽、咳痰、胸痛、虚弱、体重减轻、发热、寒战和夜间出汗。

8．Read the text and fill in the sheet with proper information.

Reading Prompts	
Items	**Your Answers**
1）*Identify the medical terms concerning* **TB** *and group them according to your understanding.*	
2）*Identify the* **adjectives** *used in* "**Diagnosis**" *and explain what conditions they describe.*	
3）*Identify the* **conjunctions** *used in* "**Quality of Life**" *and point out the logical relation each of them indicates.*（**QoL**）	
4）*Identify the* **verbs** *used in* **Exercise 3** *and point out the changes of verb tenses.*	
5）*Identify the* **typical sentence patterns.**（*the whole article*）	
6）*Identify the* **topic sentence** *and the* **supporting sentences in paragraph 1 in** "**Management**".	

Title: _____

The human immunodeficiency virus (HIV) targets the immune system and weakens people's defense against many infections and some types of cancer. As the virus destroys and impairs the function of immune cells, infected individuals gradually become immunodeficient.

The most advanced stage of HIV infection is acquired immunodeficiency syndrome (AIDS), which can take many years to develop if not treated, depending on the individual. AIDS is defined by the development of certain cancers, infections or other severe long term clinical manifestations.

The symptoms of HIV vary depending on the stage of infection. Though people living with HIV tend to be most infectious in the first few months after being infected, many are unaware of their status until the later stages. In the first few weeks after initial infection, people may experience no symptoms or an influenza-like illness including fever, headache, rash or sore throat.

As the infection progressively weakens the immune system, they can develop other signs and symptoms, such as swollen lymph nodes, weight loss, fever, diarrhea and cough. Without treatment, they could also develop severe illnesses such as tuberculosis, cryptococcal meningitis, severe bacterial infections, and cancers such as lymphomas and Kaposi's sarcoma.

HIV can be transmitted via the exchange of a variety of body fluids from infected people, such as blood, breast milk, semen and vaginal secretions. HIV can also be transmitted from a mother to her child during pregnancy and delivery. Individuals cannot become infected through ordinary day-to-day contact such as kissing, hugging, shaking hands, or sharing personal objects, food or water.

It is important to note that people with HIV who are taking antiretroviral therapy (ART) and are virally suppressed do not transmit HIV to their sexual partners. Early access to ART and remaining on treatment is therefore critical not only to improve the health of people with HIV but also to prevent HIV transmission.

HIV continues to be a major global public health issue, having claimed almost a population of 33 million lives with it so far. However, with increasing access to effective HIV prevention, diagnosis, treatment and care, including for opportunistic infections, HIV infection has become a manageable chronic health condition, enabling people living with HIV to lead long and healthy lives.

As a result of concerted international efforts to respond to HIV, coverage of services has been steadily increasing. In 2019, 68% of adults and 53% of children living with HIV globally were receiving lifelong ART.

A great majority (85%) of pregnant and breastfeeding women living with HIV also have received ART, which not only protects their health, but also ensures prevention of HIV transmission to their newborns.

By June 2020, 26 million people were accessing antiretroviral therapy, marking a 2.4% increase from an estimate of 25.4 million at the end of 2019. By comparison, treatment coverage increased by an estimated 4.8% between January and June of 2019.

The number of new people starting treatment is far below expectation due to the reduction in HIV-testing and treatment initiation and antiretroviral (ARV) disruptions in 2019. By the end of 2020, testing and treatment rates showed steady but variable recovery. However, success has been variable by region, country and population—not everyone is able to access HIV testing, treatment and care.

Interventions will need to focus on the populations left behind: key population groups and their sexual partners accounted for over 62% of all new HIV infections globally among the age group 15 – 49 years in 2019.

WHO defines key populations as people in populations who are at increased HIV risk in all countries and regions. Key populations include men who have sex with men, people who inject drugs, people in prisons and other closed settings, sex workers and their clients, and transgender people.

Increased HIV vulnerability is often associated with legal and social factors, which increases exposure to risk situations and creates barriers to accessing effective, quality and affordable HIV prevention, testing and treatment services. Prioritizing key populations in the HIV response with appropriate interventions would have the biggest impact on the epidemic and reduce new infections.

In addition, given their life circumstances, a range of other populations may be particularly vulnerable, and at increased risk of HIV infection, such as adolescent girls and young women in southern and eastern Africa and indigenous peoples in some communities.

HIV can be diagnosed through rapid diagnostic tests that can provide same-day results. HIV self-tests are increasingly available and provide an effective and acceptable alternative way to increase access to people who are not reached for HIV testing through facility-based services. Rapid test and self-tests have greatly facilitated diagnosis and linkage with treatment and care.

There is no cure for HIV infection. However, effective prevention interventions are available: preventing mother-to-child-transmission, male and female condom use, harm reduction interventions, pre-exposure prophylaxis, post exposure prophylaxis, voluntary medical male circumcision and antiretroviral drugs which can control the virus and help prevent onward transmission to other people.

Science is moving at a fast pace, and there have been two people who have achieved a "functional cure" by undergoing a bone marrow transplant for cancer with re-infusion of new CD4 T cells that are unable to be infected with HIV. However, neither a cure nor a vaccine is available to treat and protect all people currently living with or at risk of HIV.

(Extracted from https://www.who.int)

Exercises

1. Read the article and write a possible title for it.

2. Answer the following questions according to the passage.

1) What are the symptoms of HIV?

2) How is HIV transmitted?

3) What are the advantages of ART for woman with HIV?

4) Who do the key populations cover?

5) How can HIV be prevented?

UNIT 5 Surgery

Surgery is the branch of medicine concerned with the treatment of injuries, diseases, and other disorders by manual and instrumental means. Some of the most common surgical operations include appendectomy, breast biopsy, carotid endarterectomy, cataract surgery, and cesarean section (also called C-section).

Part I Intensive Reading

Acute Appendicitis

The vermiform appendix, approximately 8 to 10 cm long in adults, is a tubular structure attached to the base of the cecum at the confluence of the colic bands, which is always regarded as a degenerated organ. Acute inflammation of this structure is called acute appendicitis.

Epidemiology

Acute appendicitis is one of the most common acute surgical abdominal emergencies. Acute appendicitis occurs at a rate of about 90 to 100 patients per 100,000 inhabitants per year in developed countries. More than 250,000 appendectomies are performed each year in the US; however, the incidence is lower in populations where a high-fiber diet is consumed. The peak incidence usually occurs in the second or third decade of life, and the disease is less common at both extremes of age. Geographical differences are reported, with lifetime risks for appendicitis of 9% in the USA, and 1.8% in Africa.

A male preponderance exists, with a male to female ratio of 1 : 1 to 3 : 1. The overall lifetime risk is 9% for males and 6% for females. A difference in diagnostic error rate ranges from 12%-23% for men and 24%-42% for women. These values are a mean of the world experience, including the less advanced medical services. Most of patients are of white skin colors (74%) and is very rare in black skin color (5%). While the clinical diagnosis may be straightforward in patients who present with classic signs and symptoms, atypical presentations may result in diagnostic confusion and delay in treatment.

Mechanisms/Pathophysiology

- Obstruction

There is good evidence that if complete obstruction of the lumen occurs, appendicitis is likely to follow, usually by fecolith, fibrous band or even lymphoid hyperplasia. In clinical work, there are occasions when, for example, a cecal carcinoma obstructing the mouth of the appendix is associated with acute appendicitis. The proposed mechanism is distension and increased pressure, with consequent interference with circulation, ischemia of appendicular tissue, and invasion by bacteria. Although several infectious agents are known to trigger or be associated with appendicitis, the full range of specific causes remains unknown. Recent theories focus on infections, genetic factors, and environmental influences.

- Infection

Some investigators suggest that a viral infection could induce mucosal ulceration, which is followed by secondary bacterial invasion.

- Genetics

Although no defined gene has been identified, the risk of appendicitis is roughly three times higher in members of families with a positive history for appendicitis than in those with no family history.

- Environment

Environmental factors can play a part since studies report a predominantly seasonal presentation during the summer.

Diagnosis

The diagnosis of appendicitis can be challenging even in the most experienced hands and is predominantly a clinical one. Accurate anamnesis and physical exam are important to prevent unnecessary surgery and avoid complications. The probability of appendicitis depends on patient age, clinical setting and symptoms.

The overall accuracy for diagnosing acute appendicitis is approximately 80%, which corresponds to a mean false-negative appendectomy rate of 20%. Diagnostic accuracy varies by sex, with a range of 78% – 92% in male and 58% – 85% in female patients.

Diagnosis of acute appendicitis relies on a thorough history and examination. Abdominal pain is the primary presenting complaint of patients with acute appendicitis. Typically, the patient describes a periumbilical colicky pain, which intensifies during the first 24 hours, becoming constant and sharp, and migrates to the right iliac fossa. Nausea, vomiting and anorexia occur in varying degrees and are usually present in more than 50% of cases. A failure to recognize other presentations of acute appendicitis will lead to a delay in diagnosis and increased patient morbidity. Patients with a retrocecal appendix or those presenting in the later months of pregnancy may have pain limited to the right flank or costovertebral angle. Male patients with a retrocecal appendix may complain of right testicular pain. Pelvic or retroileal locations of an inflamed appendix will refer to the pelvis, rectum, adnexa, or rarely, the left lower quadrant. Suprapubic pain and urinary frequency may predominate.

Abdominal examination reveals localized tenderness and muscular rigidity after localization of the pain to the right iliac fossa. Patients often find that movement exacerbates the pain, and if they are asked to cough, the pain will often be localized to the right iliac fossa. Percussion tenderness and rebound tenderness are the most reliable clinical findings indicating a diagnosis of acute appendicitis. Loss of appetite, constipation and nausea are often present. The patient is often flushed, with a dry tongue and an associated bad breath. The presence of pyrexia (up to 38°C) with tachycardia is common. This classic presentation can be influenced by the age of the patient and anatomical position of the appendix.

Patients at the extremes of the age spectrum can present diagnostic difficulty because of non-specific presentation, often with subtle clinical signs. Infants and young children often seem withdrawn and elderly people may present with confusion.

No specific diagnostic test for appendicitis exists, but the judicious use of simple urine and blood tests, particularly inflammatory response variables, should allow exclusion of other pathologies and provide additional evidence to support a clinical diagnosis of appendicitis.

Radiological tests can be used to aid the diagnosis of acute appendicitis, mainly ultrasonography and computed tomography scanning, which should be done only in patients in whom a clinical and laboratory diagnosis of appendicitis cannot be made. Although ultrasonography seems to be less accurate than computed tomography scanning, it can be used as a primary imaging modality for avoiding the disadvantages of computed tomography, especially patient preparation, contrast material administration, and radiation exposure. In children, ultrasound may be preferred over computed tomography scan in order to limit radiation exposure.

Management

Appropriate resuscitation followed by expedient appendectomy is the treatment of choice. Early acute appendicitis is generally managed with surgery and prophylactic antibiotics to minimize the risk of surgical site infection. If no perforation or focal peritonitis is encountered, there is generally no need for continuation of antibiotics after surgery because the main infectious source has been removed. For perforated appendicitis, appendectomy should be performed and systemic antibiotics continued for 5 to 7 days or until fever and leukocytosis have resolved. Escherichia coli and Bacteroides fragilis are the main organisms isolated in acute simple and perforated appendicitis. Usually, after the first 36 hours from the onset of symptoms, the average rate of perforation is between 16% and 36%. However, this is significantly increased in elderly people and young children, in whom the rate can be up to 97% usually because of a delay in diagnosis. Appendectomy is a relatively safe procedure with a mortality rate for non-perforated appendicitis of 0.8 per 1000. The immediate starting of intravenous antibiotics should be used once a diagnosis of appendicitis is made and no facilities for appendectomy are available. The mortality and morbidity are related to the stage of disease and increase in cases of perforation; mortality after perforation is 5.1 per 1000. Non-operative management is primary antibiotic treatment of simple inflamed appendicitis.

However, for patients in whom appendectomy are not performed during the acute presentation, an interval appendectomy can follow 6 weeks to 3 months after the patient has recovered from the initial event. Although the need for this subsequent operation remains somewhat controversial, different studies have reported a high recurrence rate, supporting strongly considering subsequent appendectomy. Besides, there are new surgical technologies. Single-incision laparoscopic surgery and low-cost single-incision techniques have been described recently and can be done with inexpensive equipment and routine devices, leading to satisfactory functional and cosmetic results. There has been some debate regarding the best surgical approach for appendectomy: laparoscopic versus open. Results from multiple randomized controlled trials have been reported, and a recent review of the literature favors the laparoscopic approach because of better postoperative outcomes including lower rate of SSI, shorter length of stay, and faster return to work. Although the direct costs, operative time, and incidence of intra-abdominal abscesses may be higher, the laparoscopic approach is currently the standard of care given the reported benefits after surgery.

Quality of Life

If patients are treated in a timely fashion, the prognosis is good. Wound infection and intra-abdominal abscess are potential complications associated with appendectomy. Laparoscopic appendectomy has been shown to decrease the incidence of overall complications.

Prevention

Appendicitis occurs when the appendix becomes so severely inflamed or infected that it causes pain, discomfort, and requires treatment that most likely includes surgical removal. Unfortunately, there are currently no known methods for preventing the painful and potentially fatal inflammation. Some lifestyle factors may appear to reduce chances of getting appendicitis, such as eating a high-fiber diet, exercise, vitamin supplements, and so on. Populations with diets high in fiber have fewer cases of appendicitis. So, it would not be a stretch to assume that there are appendicitis foods to eat that could help avoid that medical condition.

- High-fiber diet

Eating a diet high in fiber may be one of the best ways to possibly avoid appendicitis. Exactly why fiber can help avoid appendicitis has yet to be confirmed by science, but there is a theory that it has to do with fiber's effects on the body. Fiber helps with the digestion process by allowing food to pass through the body more smoothly. Instead of breaking down and absorbing dietary fiber, the body sends it along the digestive tract in whole. This not only helps to get the digestible nutrients to where they need to go, but it also helps move the waste through the intestines and out of the body. The idea is that, along with the waste, bacteria and other harmful elements that may cause appendicitis will quickly exit the body and not get a foothold that will lead to inflammation and infection. Foods that contain fiber include whole grains, fruits, vegetables, beans, legumes, nuts, seeds, oats pulses, apples, oranges, carrots, tomato, cucumber, spinach etc. Besides, supplements can be used in order to bring the amount of fiber up in your body, such as vitamins A and D. Vitamin A can help raise the white blood cell count, which helps battle infections throughout the body and vitamin D is a good vitamin for fighting bacteria.

- Balanced diet

Along with adding more fiber to diet, eating a more balanced diet may also lower chances of appendicitis. Eating a diet low in saturated and trans fats, processed foods, and high in fiber, can reduce chances of general illness and infection that may lead to an infection of appendix. While this will not prevent appendicitis, the healthier people are, the less chance it will occur.

• Exercise

Exercise is good for overall health, including reducing the risk of cardiovascular disease, diabetes and some cancers. In this case, it may also be good for appendix. Exercise does two very important things. Regular exercise can keep the body healthy, making it harder for disease, infections, and inflammation to take hold in the body. Fewer infections for the body mean a reduced chance of the appendix becoming infected.

(Extracted from *The BMJ*)

Vocabulary

appendix	[ə'pendɪks]	*n.* 阑尾
cecum	['siːkəm]	*n.* 盲肠
confluence	['kɒnfluəns]	*n.* 聚集；合并
hyperplasia	[ˌhaɪpə'pleɪʒə]	*n.* 增生；畸形生长
distension	[dɪ'stenʃn]	*n.* 膨胀，扩张
ulceration	[ˌʌlsə'reɪʃn]	*n.* 溃疡形成
anamnesis	[ˌænæm'nɪsɪs]	*n.* 既往症
retrocecal	[ˌretrəʊ'sɪkəl]	*adj.* 盲肠后的
retroileal	[riːtrɔɪ'liːl]	*adj.* 回肠后位
umbilical	[ʌm'bɪlɪkl]	*adj.* 脐带的
colicky	['kɒlɪkɪ]	*adj.* 疝气痛的；腹绞痛的
constipation	[ˌkɒnstɪ'peɪʃn]	*n.* 便秘
pyrexia	[paɪ'reksɪə]	*n.* 发热；热病
tachycardia	[ˌtækɪ'kaːdɪə]	*n.* 心动过速
resuscitation	[rɪˌsʌsɪ'teɪʃn]	*n.* 复苏
prophylactic	[ˌprɒfə'læktɪk]	*adj.* 预防性的 *n.* 预防性药物
peritonitis	[ˌperɪtə'naɪtɪs]	*n.* 腹膜炎
leukocytosis	[ˌluːkəʊsaɪ'təʊsɪs]	*n.* 白细胞增多
laparoscopic	[ˌlæpərə'skɒpɪk]	*adj.* 腹腔镜检查的
abscess	['æbses]	*n.* 脓肿；脓疮

Exercises

1. Read the text and explain the following medical phrases.

1) Symptoms of acute appendicitis

2) Causes of acute appendicitis

3) Management of acute appendicitis

4) Prevention for acute appendicitis

2. Answer the following questions according to the text.

1) How does acute appendicitis influence different sexes?

2) What tests can help diagnose acute appendicitis?

3) How does a doctor diagnose acute appendicitis?

4) What kind of diet habit could be beneficial to prevent appendicitis?

3. Fill in the blanks with the proper forms of the given words.

| innervation | colicky | constipation | confuse | anatomy |
| periumbilical | perforate | iliac fossa | appendicitis | migrate |

Abdominal pain is the primary complaint of patients with acute 1)_____.
The diagnostic sequence of 2)_____ central abdominal pain followed by
vomiting with migration of the pain to the right 3)_____ area was first
described by Murphy but may only be present in 50% of patients. Typically, the
patient describes a colicky pain, which intensifies during the first 24 hours,
becoming constant and sharp, and migrates to the right 4)_____. The initial
pain represents a referred pain resulting from the visceral 5)_____ of the
midgut, and the localized pain is caused by involvement of the parietal peritoneum
after progression of the inflammatory process. Loss of appetite is often a
predominant feature, and 6)_____ and nausea are often present. Profuse
vomiting may indicate development of generalized peritonitis after 7)_____ but
is rarely a major feature in simple appendicitis. A meta-analysis of the symptoms
and signs associated with a presentation of acute appendicitis is unable to identify
any one diagnostic finding but shows that a 8)_____ of pain is associated with
a diagnosis of acute appendicitis. This classic presentation can be influenced by
the age of the patient and 9)_____ position of the appendix. Patients at the
extremes of the age spectrum can present diagnostic difficulty because of non-
specific presentation, often with subtle clinical signs. Infants and young children
often seem withdrawn, and elderly people may present with 10)_____. A high

index of suspicion for acute appendicitis is needed in such patients.

4. **Study the bold-faced words in each of the following sentences and imitate the particular way of writing.**

Mentor Sentence：

☆ In morbidly obese patients, bariatric surgery **can be an effective means of** weight loss.

Imitation Sentence：

☆ Parenteral vaccination **can be an effective means of** inducing protective mucosal responses.

1）**There is good evidence that** if complete obstruction of the lumen occurs, appendicitis is likely to follow, usually by fecolith, fibrous band or even lymphoid hyperplasia.

Answer：**There is good evidence that** _____

_____

2）**The risk of** appendicitis **is roughly** three **times higher in members of** families with a positive history for appendicitis **than** in those with no family history.

Answer：**The risk of** _____ **is roughly** _____ **times higher in members of** _____ **than** _____

_____

3）Abdominal pain **is the primary complaint of patients with** acute appendicitis.

Answer：_____ **is the primary complaint of patients with** _____

4）**There has been some debate regarding** the best surgical approach **for** appendectomy: laparoscopic versus open.

Answer：**There has been some debate regarding** _____ **for**

_____

5. **Match the following statements with the corresponding sections in the text.**

Epidemiology：_____   Management：_____

Mechanisms/Pathophysiology：_____   Quality of Life：_____

Diagnosis：_____   Prevention：_____

A. Appendicitis is likely to follow complete obstruction of the lumen.

B. Besides, recent theories focus on infections, genetic factors, and environmental influences.

C. Diagnosis of acute appendicitis relies on a thorough history and examination.

D. Abdominal pain is the primary complaint of patients with acute appendicitis, as well as loss of appetite, constipation and nausea.

E. Appendicitis treatment usually involves surgery to remove the inflamed appendix, usually by laparoscopic appendectomy or open appendectomy.

F. Acute appendicitis is one of the most common acute surgical abdominal emergencies.

G. The peak incidence usually occurs in the second or third decade of life.

H. Most studies show a slight male predominance.

I. There are currently no known methods for preventing the painful and potentially fatal inflammation.

J. Some lifestyle factors may appear to reduce chances of getting appendicitis.

K. Radiological tests and the judicious use of simple urine, blood tests, and inflammatory response variables can be used to aid the diagnosis.

L. If patients are treated in a timely fashion, the prognosis is good.

M. Non-operative management is primary antibiotic treatment of simple inflamed appendicitis or no facilities for appendectomy.

6. Read the introduction in the box and finish the exercises after it.

> In composition, **cause and effects** is a method of paragraph development in which a writer analyzes the reasons for—and/or the consequences of—an action, event or a decision. The cause-and-effect pattern may be used to identify one or more causes followed by one or more effects or results. A cause states why something happens. An effects states a result or outcome. At times, **a single cause leads to several effects**. Other times, **several causes contribute to a single effect**. A causal chain is a sequence of events in which any one event in the chain causes the next one, leading up to a final effect.

1) Circle the single effects and underline the causes.

Appendicitis happens when the inside of your appendix is blocked. Appendicitis may be caused by various infections such as virus, bacteria, or parasites in digestive tract. Or it may happen when the tube that joins large intestine and appendix is blocked or trapped by stool. Sometimes tumors can cause appendicitis.

2) Reorder the following sentences to make an effective paragraph.

A. Typically, the patient describes a periumbilical colicky pain, and the pain migrates to the right iliac fossa.

B. Patients often find that movement or cough exacerbates the pain.

C. This classic presentation can be influenced by the age of the patient and anatomical position of the appendix.

D. Diagnosis of acute appendicitis relies on a thorough history and examination.

E. Besides, loss of appetite, constipation and nausea often present.

F. The patient is often flushed with a dry tongue and an associated bad breath.

Answer：__ __ __ __ __ __

7. **Translate the Chinese paragraph below into English.**

急性阑尾炎是外科常见病,居各种急腹症首位。转移性右下腹痛及阑尾点压痛、反跳痛为常见临床表现,常伴有呕吐、发热等。急性阑尾炎发病与饮食习惯、便秘和遗传等因素有关。虽然基因的影响尚未明确,但有家族史的患者数量多于没有家族病史的患者数量。

8. **Read the text and fill in the sheet with proper information.**

Reading Prompts	
Items	**Your Answers**
1) *Identify the medical terms concerning **acute appendicitis** and group them according to your understanding.*	
2) *Identify the **adjectives** used in "**Epidemiology**" and explain what conditions they describe.*	
3) *Identify the **conjunctions** used in "**Mechanisms/Pathophysiology**" and point out the logical relation each of them indicates.*	
4) *Identify the **verbs** used in "**Balanced Diet**" and point out the changes of verb tenses.*	
5) *Identify the **typical sentence patterns**. (**the whole article**)*	
6) *Identify the **topic sentence** and the **supporting sentences** in "**High-fiber diet**".*	

Title: _____

By the middle of the nineteenth century, post-operative sepsis infection accounted for the death of almost half of the patients undergoing major surgery. A common report by surgeons was: operation successful but the patient died. Now, it is known that bacteria are everywhere, and some are good for us while others are harmful. Bacteria, viruses and other microorganisms that cause disease are called pathogens. To protect patients from harmful bacteria and other pathogens during medical procedures, healthcare providers use aseptic technique.

Aseptic technique means using practices and procedures to prevent contamination from pathogens. It involves applying the strictest rules to minimize the risk of infection. Healthcare workers use aseptic technique in surgery rooms, clinics, outpatient care centers and other health care settings.

When mentioning aseptic technique, there is an important person who can not be forgotten—Hungarian obstetrician Ignaz Philipp Semmelweis, who was born July 1, 1818 and died August 13, 1865. While working at the maternity department of the Vienna General Hospital in 1846, he was concerned with the rate of puerperal fever (also called childbed fever) among the women who gave birth there. This was often a deadly condition.

The rate for puerperal fever was five times higher in the ward that was staffed by male doctors and medical students and lower in the ward staffed by midwives. Why should this be? He tried eliminating various possibilities, from the position of giving birth to eliminating a walk-through by a priest after patients died. These had no effect.

In 1847, Dr. Ignaz Semmelweis's close friend, Jakob Kolletschka, cut his finger while doing an autopsy. Kolletschka soon died of symptoms like those of puerperal fever. This led Semmelweis to note that the doctors and medical students often performed autopsies, while the midwives did not. He theorized that particles from the cadavers were responsible for transmitting the disease.

He instituted washing hands and instruments with soap and chlorine. At this time, the existence of germs was not generally known or accepted. The miasma theory of disease was the standard one and chlorine would remove any ill vapors. The cases of puerperal fever dropped dramatically when doctors were made to wash after doing an autopsy.

He lectured publicly about his results in 1850. However, his observations and results were no match for the entrenched belief that disease was due to an imbalance of humors or spread by miasmas. It was also an irritating task that put blame on spreading disease on the doctors themselves. Semmelweis spent 14 years developing and promoting his ideas, including publishing a poorly reviewed book in 1861. In 1865, he suffered a nervous breakdown and was committed to an insane asylum where he soon died from blood poisoning.

Only after Dr. Semmelweis's death was the germ theory of disease developed, and he is now recognized as a pioneer of antiseptic policy and prevention of nosocomial disease.

Handwashing between patients is now recognized as the best way to prevent spreading illness in health care settings. It is still difficult to get full compliance from doctors, nurses and other members of the health care team. Using sterile technique and sterile instruments in surgery has had better success.

There are four chief aspects of the aseptic technique: barriers, patient equipment and preparation, environmental controls, and contact guidelines. Each plays an important role in infection prevention during a medical procedure.

Barriers protect the patient from the transfer of pathogens from a healthcare worker, from the environment, or from both. Some barriers used in aseptic technique include sterile gloves, sterile gowns, masks for the patient and healthcare provider and sterile drapes.

Sterile barriers are those that have not touched a contaminated surface. They are specially packaged and cleaned items. Healthcare workers put them on or use them in specific ways that minimize exposure to germs.

Healthcare providers also use sterile equipment and sterile instruments. To further protect the patient, they apply cleansing and bacteria-killing preparations to the patient's skin before a procedure.

Maintaining a sterile environment requires keeping doors closed during an operation. Only necessary health personnel should be at the procedure. The more people present, the more opportunities for harmful bacteria to cause contamination.

Once healthcare providers have sterile barriers on, they should only touch other sterile items. They should avoid touching nonsterile items at all costs.

A common procedure that carries a risk for infection is inserting a urinary catheter. These catheters drain urine from the bladder and are associated with catheter-associated urinary tract infections. When healthcare providers insert a catheter, they demonstrate all four aseptic techniques in action. For example, they wear sterile gloves; they open sterile packaging that contains the sterile catheter; they prepare the patient's skin with a special solution with only one or two providers and the patient in the room; healthcare providers take great care not to touch any nonsterile surface with the hand that advances the catheter into the patient's urethra. If even one part of the aseptic technique is missed during catheter insertion, the patient can easily get an infection.

(Extracted from https://www.thoughtco.com)

Exercises

1. **Read the article and write a possible title for it.**

2. **Answer the following questions according to the passage.**

   1) What would happen to the patients after operation in the 19th century?

   2) How did Semmelweis discover the importance of washing hands?

   3) Why did people disagree with Semmelweis then?

   4) What happened to Semmelweis's theory after his death?

   5) What are the four chief aspects of aseptic technique?

UNIT 6 Reproductive Medicine

Reproductive system disease consists of diseases and disorders that affect the human reproductive system. Reproductive disorders include abnormal hormone production of ovaries or testes, and that of other endocrine glands such as pituitary, thyroid, or adrenals. Such diseases can also be caused by genetic or congenital abnormalities, infections, tumors, or disorders of unknown cause.

Part I   Intensive Reading

Polycystic Ovary Syndrome

Polycystic ovary/ovarian syndrome (PCOS) is a set of symptoms related to an imbalance of hormones that can affect women and girls of reproductive age. PCOS is most often diagnosed by the presence of two of the three following criteria: chronic anovulation, hyperandrogenism and poly cystic ovaries on ultrasonography.

Epidemiology

PCOS is the most common endocrinopathy of women of reproductive age. Its high prevalence has attracted significant public attention. PCOS is a complex endocrine condition, due to its heterogeneity and uncertainty about its etiology. It is recommended that the diagnostic criteria for PCOS should comprise the concomitant presence of anovulation and evidence of hyperandrogenemia—biochemical, clinical (hirsutism/acne) or both—but without reference to ovarian morphology.

In order to provide a more inclusive definition of the syndrome, the report of a meeting of experts at a joint meeting held in Rotterdam in 2003 proposed that the presence of two of the three criteria, chronic anovulation, hyperandrogenism and polycystic ovaries on ultrasonography, would be sufficient for PCOS diagnosis. Nevertheless, disagreements remained as clearly illustrated in a study conducted in 2005, in which it was found that the majority of gynecologists considered that polycystic ovaries on ultrasound was an essential tool for PCOS diagnosis, whereas the endocrinologist's view was more focused on hirsutism and anovulation.

Since PCOS is a very common disorder (the prevalence ranges from 6% to 20% depending on the criteria used), it would be helpful to have unity about the diagnostic criteria.

Mechanisms/Pathophysiology

PCOS can be found from early infancy to puberty, based on predisposing environmental influences and genetic factors. There is some evidence that PCOS may partly depend on genetic factors. However, it is unlikely that PCOS represents a single gene defect and it is more likely to be polygenic or oligogenic. On the other hand, low birth weight and fetal exposure to androgens may contribute to the development of PCOS. In addition, low birth weight is particularly associated with insulin resistance and obesity in adulthood. It is suggested that the clinical features of PCOS may develop as a consequence of genetically determined hypersecretion of androgens by the ovary starting at puberty or very likely long before puberty, so that typical clinical and biochemical characteristics of PCOS may become expressed as a consequence of exposure to androgen excess at or before puberty. Through its effects on programming of the hypothalamo-pituitary unit, hyperandrogenism in fetal life favors excess luteinizing hormone (LH) secretion and leads to the development of abdominal obesity and consequent insulin resistance. Altered steroid negative feedback regulation of LH together with the compensatory hyperinsulinemia due to insulin resistance may disrupt ovulatory function, causing anovulation. Intrauterine factors and possible changes in the intrauterine environment may also play a role in the happening of PCOS.

Diagnosis

Polycystic means "many cysts". A main feature of PCOS is that eggs are not released from the ovaries. Instead, fluid builds up around the eggs, forming sacs (cysts). Healthcare practitioners will typically diagnose a woman (adult female) as having PCOS if she has at least two of the following features:

□ *Excess male hormones (androgens)—evidence of this may include a high blood testosterone level, for example, or symptoms such as acne (sometimes severe) and excess hair growth, which can be on the face, stomach and/or back.*

□ *Problems with ovulation—this may include having no menstrual periods, irregular menstrual cycles, or infertility.*

□ *Ultrasound results that show large ovaries with many small follicles that look like cysts (No ultrasound may be needed if a woman has both of the first two features.)*

The underlying causes of PCOS are not well understood, but it is believed that an imbalance of sex hormones and insulin resistance are the main problems. These problems can result in a defined group of signs, symptoms and complications, such as excess facial and body hair, weight gain, irregular menstrual periods, infertility, and increased risk of diabetes and heart disease.

- Testosterone

Testosterone is the main circulating active androgen, and the total serum testosterone concentration is the first-line recommendation for assessing androgen excess in women.

- Sex hormone-binding globulin

Low Sex hormone-binding globulin (SHBG) has shown excellent diagnostic accuracy for the diagnosis of PCOS, even superior to measurements of serum androgen concentrations, and low SHBG is a surrogate marker of insulin resistance and androgen excess that predicts the susceptibility to develop metabolic syndrome and gestational diabetes in women with PCOS.

- Vitamin D

Deficiency of vitamin D is very common in women with PCOS, particularly in those with obesity. It has been suggested that vitamin D status may contribute to the development of the metabolic disturbances associated with PCOS, chiefly insulin resistance and glucose intolerance states.

- Obesity of PCOS

Obesity, particularly the abdominal phenotype, is undoubtedly a useful clinical predictor of metabolic abnormalities which can be detected in the early stages of PCOS and, sometimes, it even precedes its development. It is also very frequent in PCOS. The distribution of fat to abdominal area is unlikely to be the entire explanation for the metabolic abnormalities observed in PCOS women. However, this distribution together with the amount of body fat contributes significantly to the expression and severity of PCOS. It has been demonstrated that the adipose tissue of

PCOS has an aberrant function. In particular, adipocytes from women with PCOS are hypertrophic and there is an impaired activity of the sympathetic system in their abdominal fat.

- Sleep disorders in PCOS

Limited available data suggest that obstructive sleep apnea (OSA) is more common in obese PCOS women both in adolescence and during reproductive years, compared with the general population. Overall, sleep disordered breathing and daytime sleepiness appear to be two to three-fold increase in obese PCOS patients. Alternatively, normal weight women with PCOS do not seem to have an increased risk of sleep disorders. Androgen excess might be associated with the presence of OSA in PCOS. The presence of OSA increases cardiometabolic risk in PCOS similarly to non-PCOS women, whereas treatment of OSA with continuous positive airway pressure is associated with improvement in cardiometabolic dysfunction of PCOS. Nevertheless, it seems wise at this moment to screen sleep disorders by clinical questionnaires in obese women with PCOS.

- CV risk factors

There is an increased prevalence of cardiovascular (CV) risk factors in women with PCOS. This is reflected in impaired endothelial function at an early age. Besides the early functional impairment of the vascular wall, the morphologic signs of early atherogenesis are highly prevalent in young women with PCOS. Whether the risk translates into increased CV morbidity and mortality has not yet been fully elucidated as appropriate long-term prospective studies are lacking. The data on CV events in PCOS women are inconsistent due to different criteria used to retrospectively confirm the diagnosis of PCOS. Some of the studies including very high numbers of women point towards an increase in either CV morbidity or even mortality in women with irregular menses, or increased incidence of stroke in PCOS women from the UK. A prospective study on 32 PCOS patients followed for 21 years did not confirm these data. A large study has shown an association between menstrual irregularity and increased age-adjusted risk for CV mortality, which lost significance after adjusting for BMI, while the recent meta-analysis has reported a twofold relative risk for arterial disease irrespective of BMI.

Management

This section summarizes some major therapeutic choices in the treatment of PCOS.

- Bariatric surgery

In morbidly obese patients, bariatric surgery can be an effective means of weight loss and most women may resolve PCOS signs and symptoms. Bariatric surgery may in fact prevent or reverse the metabolic syndrome and may also have reproductive benefits.

- Insulin sensitizers and other antidiabetic drugs

Metformin is the most widely used insulin sensitizer drug to treat women with insulin resistance and PCOS. The benefits of metformin treatment are believed to target both cardiometabolic disorders and the reproductive abnormalities. Thiazolidinediones (TZDs) are another class of insulin sensitizing drugs that have been studied in women with PCOS. Pioglitazone and rosiglitazone, the two currently available TZDs, have been shown to be effective in improving some metabolic, hormonal as well as reproductive parameters of PCOS.

- Use of oral contraceptives and progestins

COCs (Combined oral contraceptives) have an important place in the management of both menstrual disorders and androgen excess symptoms. Progestins, usually given cyclically, also have a role in the management of menstrual dysfunction. Although COCs remain the mainstay of the pharmacological therapy of PCOS, even low dose pills may contribute to an increased risk of metabolic abnormalities, CV events and venous thromboembolism.

- Use of anti-androgens

Anti-androgen drugs may be used alone or combined with another anti-androgen, an insulinsensitizer or with an oral contraceptive pill. The combined treatments are generally more effective than one drug alone. In particular, a combination of an anti-androgen and COCs with metformin may lead to more beneficial metabolic effects than monotherapy with either an anti-androgen or a COC. There are sufficient data to confirm that low doses of anti-androgens are as effective as high doses of anti-androgens, so the lowest effective dose of an anti-androgen agent should be used to avoid dose-related side effects and reduce costs.

Quality of Life

Available data show that PCOS status may have significant negative consequences on the psychological wellbeing. Most cohort studies have demonstrated that the prevalence of both anxiety and depression may be higher than expected. Another study showed that, a higher lifetime incidence of depressive episodes, social phobia, and eating disorders, and, dramatically, of suicide attempts does occur. A recent study has found that depression was related more to infertility while anxiety more to excess weight or obesity, whereas other studies have reported that obesity was also independently related to depression. Interestingly one prospective study reported that, after 6 months of COCs use, the PCO syndrome quality scores on body hair and menstrual problems were significantly improved along with a clinical improvement in hirsutism and menstrual irregularity, although depression and anxiety mean scores and depression rates did not show a significant change. Conversely, in obese PCOS women, weight loss has been found to improve depression and quality of life.

Prevention

Lifestyle modification, including diet and exercise, is considered a cornerstone of the management of women with PCOS presenting with obesity. On one hand, dietary advice is the major component of lifestyle modification, especially in obese patients. There is little evidence suggesting that the composition of the diet may influence the final outcomes, since weight loss improved the presentation of PCOS regardless of dietary composition in most studies. On the other hand, only a few studies have addressed whether exercise training and specific exercise programs exert beneficial effects on PCOS. Physical exercise may improve fitness, CV, hormonal, reproductive and psychological parameters in patients with PCOS. The type, intensity, and frequency of exercise required for treating PCOS are far from being established.

(Extracted from *European Journal of Endocrinology*)

Vocabulary

anovulation	[æˌnɒvjʊˈleɪʃn]	*n.* 排卵停止
acne	[ˈækni]	*n.* 痤疮
hyperandrogenism	[haɪpəˈrændrɒdʒɪnɪzəm]	*n.* 雄性激素过多症
hirsutism	[ˈhɜːsjʊˌtɪzəm]	*n.* 多毛症
oligogenic	[ɒlɪɡəˈdʒenɪk]	*adj.* 寡基因的
androgen	[ˈændrədʒən]	*n.* 雄激素
ovulatory	[ˈɒvjʊlətrɪ]	*adj.* 排卵的
intrauterine	[ˌɪntrəˈjuːtəraɪn]	*adj.* 子宫内的
testosterone	[teˈstɒstərəʊn]	*n.* 睾酮
menstrual	[ˈmenstrʊəl]	*adj.* 月经的
globulin	[ˈɡlɒbjʊlɪn]	*n.* 球蛋白
gestational	[dʒeˈsteɪʃənəl]	*adj.* 妊娠期的
glucose	[ˈɡluːkəʊs]	*n.* 葡萄糖
adipose	[ˈædɪpəʊs]	*adj.* 用于贮存脂肪的
aberrant	[æˈberənt]	*adj.* 异常的
contraceptive	[ˌkɒntrəˈseptɪv]	*n.* 避孕药

| progestin | [prəʊˈdʒestɪn] | n. 黄体酮 |
| venous | [ˈviːnəs] | adj. 静脉的 |

Exercises

1. Read the text and explain the following medical phrases.

1) Criteria of PCOS

2) Causes of PCOS

3) Biomarkers of PCOS

4) Treatment of PCOS

2. Answer the following questions according to the text.

1) What are the signs and symptoms of PCOS?

2) What are the side effects of using oral contraceptives in treating PCOS?

3) What can be used together with anti-androgen drugs to treat PCOS?

4) How can bariatric surgery be used in treating PCOS?

3. Fill in the blanks with the proper forms of the given words.

| morbid | atherogenesis | mortal | artery | menses |
| cardiovascular | diagnose | endothelial | stroke | follow |

There is an increased prevalence of 1)＿＿＿＿ (CV) risk factors in women with PCOS. This is reflected in impaired 2)＿＿＿＿ function at an early age. Besides the early functional impairment of the vascular wall, the morphologic signs of early 3)＿＿＿＿ are highly prevalent in young women with PCOS. Whether the risk translates into increased CV morbidity and 4)＿＿＿＿ has not yet been fully elucidated as appropriate long-term prospective studies are lacking. The data on CV events in PCOS women are inconsistent due to different criteria used to retrospectively confirm the 5)＿＿＿＿ of PCOS. Some of the studies including very high numbers of women point towards an increase in either CV 6)＿＿＿＿ and even mortality in women with irregular 7)＿＿＿＿, or increased incidence of 8)＿＿＿＿ in PCOS women. A prospective study on 32 PCOS patients being 9)＿＿＿＿ for 21 years did not confirm these data. A large study has shown an association between menstrual irregularity and increased age-adjusted risk for CV mortality, which lost significance after adjusting for BMI, while the recent meta-analysis has reported a twofold relative risk for 10)＿＿＿＿ disease irrespective of BMI.

4. Study the bold-faced words in each of the following sentences and imitate the particular way of writing.

Mentor Sentence:

☆ In morbidly obese patients, bariatric surgery **can be an effective means of** weight loss.

Imitation Sentence:

☆ Parenteral vaccination **can be an effective means of** inducing protective mucosal responses.

1) On the other hand, low birth weight and fetal exposure to androgens **may contribute to the development of** PCOS.

Answer: _____ **may contribute to the development of** _____

_____

2) Testosterone is the main circulating active androgen, and the total serum testosterone concentration **is the first-line recommendation for assessing** androgen excess in women.

Answer: _____ **is the first-line recommendation for assessing** _____

_____

3) Low SHBG **has shown excellent diagnostic accuracy for the diagnosis of** PCOS in epidemiological studies.

Answer: _____ **has shown excellent diagnostic accuracy for the diagnosis of** _____

_____

4) Obesity, particularly the abdominal phenotype, **is undoubtedly a useful clinical predictor of** metabolic abnormalities **which can be detected in the early stages of** PCOS and, sometimes, it even precedes its development.

Answer: _____ **is undoubtedly a useful clinical predictor of** _____ _____ **which can be detected in the early stages of** _____

_____

5. Match the following statements with the corresponding sections in the text.

Epidemiology:_____   Management:_____
Mechanisms/Pathophysiology: _____   Quality of Life:_____
Diagnosis:_____   Prevention:_____

A. Polycystic ovary syndrome (PCOS) is the most common ovarian disorder associated with androgen excess in women, which justifies the growing interest of endocrinologists.

B. Great efforts have been made in the last two decades to define the syndrome.

C. The presence of three different definitions for the diagnosis of PCOS reflects the phenotypic heterogeneity of the syndrome.

D. Major criteria are required for the diagnosis, which in turn identifies different phenotypes according to the combination of different criteria.

E. In addition, the relevant impact of metabolic issues, specifically insulin resistance and obesity, on the pathogenesis of PCOS, and the susceptibility to develop earlier than expected glucose intolerance states, including type 2 diabetes, have supported the notion that these aspects should be considered when defining the PCOS phenotype and planning potential therapeutic strategies in an affected subject.

F. This paper offers a critical endocrine and European perspective on the debate on the definition of PCOS and summarizes all major aspects related to etiological factors, including early life events, potentially involved in the development of the disorder.

G. Diagnostic tools of PCOS are also discussed, with emphasis on the laboratory evaluation of androgens and other potential biomarkers of ovarian and metabolic dysfunctions.

H. More research is needed to better understand disease mechanisms and to develop new treatments that reduce disease activity and progression.

I. We have also paid specific attention to the role of obesity, sleep disorders and the relevant pathogenetic aspects of cardiovascular risk factors.

J. In addition, we have discussed how to target treatment choices according to the phenotype and individual patient's needs.

K. Finally, we have suggested potential areas of translational and clinical research for the future with specific emphasis on hormonal and metabolic aspects of PCOS.

6. Read the introduction in the box and finish the exercises after it.

> In composition, **cause and effects** is a method of paragraph development in which a writer analyzes the reasons for—and/or the consequences of—an action, event or a decision. The cause-and-effect pattern may be used to identify one or more causes followed by one or more effects or results. A cause states why something happens. An effects states a result or outcome. At times, **a single cause leads to several effects**. Other times, **several causes contribute to a single effects**. A **causal chain** is a sequence of events in which any one event in the chain causes the next one, leading up to a final effects.

1) Draw the causal chain of the following paragraph.

In some cases, a woman does not make enough of the hormones needed to ovulate. When ovulation does not happen, the ovaries can develop many small fluid-filled sacs (cysts). These cysts make hormones called androgens. Androgens are a type of hormone found in abundance in men, but women normally have them in smaller amounts. Women with PCOS often have high levels of androgens. This can cause more problems with a woman's menstrual cycle and it can cause many of the symptoms of PCOS.

2) Reorder the following sentences to make an effective paragraph.

A. The high levels of insulin help stimulate the ovaries to overproduce androgen hormones, which may be the cause of PCOS in some women.

B. So, instead of having a pear shape, women with PCOS have more of an apple shape.

C. Insulin resistance can lead to hyperinsulinism or hyperinsulinemia.

D. Since the weight gain is triggered by male hormones, it is typically in the abdomen.

E. High androgen levels lead to symptoms such as body hair growth, acne, irregular periods and weight gain.

F. That is where men tend to carry weight.

Answer: __ __ __ __ __ __

7. Translate the Chinese paragraph below into English.

多囊卵巢综合征(PCOS)是一种复杂的内分泌及代谢异常疾病,常见于生育年龄的妇女,以慢性无排卵(排卵功能紊乱或丧失)和高雄激素血症(妇女体内男性激素产生过剩)为特征,主要临床表现为月经周期不规律、不孕、多毛和/或痤疮,是最常见的女性内分泌疾病。

8. Read the text and fill in the sheet with proper information.

Reading Prompts	
Items	**Your Answers**
1) *Identify the medical terms concerning* **PCOS** *and group them according to your understanding.*	

continued

Reading Prompts	
Items	**Your Answers**
2） *Identify the* **adjectives** *used in* "**Mechanisms/ Pathophysiology**" *and explain what conditions they describe.*	
3） *Identify the* **conjunctions** *used in* "**Sleep disorders in PCOS**" *and point out the logical relation each of them indicates.*	
4） *Identify the* **modal verbs** *used in* "**Use of anti- androgens**" *and point out how to use them.*	
5） *Identify the* **typical sentence patterns**. （**the whole article**）	
6） *Identify the* **topic sentence** *and the* **supporting sentences** *in* "**Obesity of PCOS**".	

Title: _____

The Nobel prize in physiology or medicine has been awarded this year to Robert G. Edwards, an English biologist who with a physician colleague, Dr. Patrick Steptoe, developed the in vitro fertilization procedure for treating human infertility.

Since the birth of the first test tube baby, Louise Brown, on July 25, 1978, some four million babies worldwide have been conceived by mixing eggs and sperm outside the body and returning the embryo to the womb to resume the normal development. The procedure overcomes many previously untreatable causes of infertility and is used in three percent of all live births in developed countries.

Research with human embryonic stem cells, made possible by Dr. Edwards's development of in vitro fertilization, has evoked a similar outcry, but so far there are no offsetting practical benefits like the birth of healthy babies to eager parents. Because of the difficulty of stem cell research, such benefits may not be seen for many years, if ever.

Dr. Edwards, a physiologist who spent much of his career at Cambridge University in England, devoted more than 20 years to solving a series of problems in getting eggs and sperm to mature and unite successfully outside the body. His colleague, Dr. Steptoe, was a gynecologist and pioneer of laparoscopic surgery, the method he used to extract eggs from the prospective mother.

Dr. Steptoe, who presumably would otherwise have shared the prize, died in 1988 (the Nobel prize is not awarded posthumously). Dr. Edwards, 85, has retired as head of research from the Bourn Hall Clinic in Cambridge, which he and Dr. Steptoe founded as one of the world's first centers for in vitro fertilization.

Because of health issues, Dr. Edwards himself was not available to reflect on his research career or the four million children alive because of his achievement. "Unfortunately he is not in a position to understand the honor he has received today," said Dr. Michael Macnamee, director of the Bourn Hall clinic and a longtime colleague of Dr. Edwards. "He remembers the past very well, but not the present."

Though in vitro fertilization is now widely accepted, the birth of the first test tube baby was greeted with intense concern that the moral order was being subverted by unnatural intervention in the mysterious process of creating a human being. Dr. Edwards was well aware of the ethical issues raised by his research and took the lead in addressing them. In parallel with defending his work in public, Dr. Edwards had to surmount one daunting problem after another in his laboratory. It sounds easy mix eggs and sperm in a Petri dish and let nature do the rest. But the opposite is the case.

At the outset of his research, Dr. Edwards wasted two years trying to get eggs to mature outside the body, based on a report that human eggs matured in 12 hours. Eventually he learned that at least 25 hours is required.

Needing a reliable supply of human eggs, he approached Dr. Steptoe at the Oldham and District General Hospital because of his expertise at retrieving unfertilized eggs from the ovary through minute incisions in the patient's skin. The two agreed to work as equals, to halt their work if danger emerged to patients or children and to ignore all religious and political criticism they deemed frivolous. The partnership lasted 20 years, until Dr. Steptoe's death.

The two began transferring fertilized eggs to the womb in 1972, assuming that the rate of implantation would be as high as with farm animals. Their hopes were dashed. At first, the hormones given the mother to induce ovulation interfered with the growth of the embryo. Drs. Edwards and Steptoe then injected mothers with extra hormones, but these turned out to induce abortions.

They persisted through more than 40 embryo transfers before obtaining their first pregnancy. Unfortunately it was ectopic and had to be aborted. Louise Brown was born from the second pregnancy.

"It required grit and determination to keep going," Dr. Macnamee said of his colleague. "But he had the conviction of his research work and he wanted to see it delivered to the people who needed it. "

Despite the ethical objections leveled at his work—some of which persist today, over the disposal of unused embryos and the high risk of multiple births—Dr. Edwards was nonetheless allowed to develop the technique over many years. "It would be very difficult to develop in vitro fertilization now because the ethical committees would have stopped his research," Dr. Macnamee said.

The ability to fertilize eggs in a dish made possible several other significant advances in reproductive technology, such as pre-implantation diagnosis of genetic diseases and the culturing of embryonic stem cells.

Dr. Edwards was keenly interested in human embryonic stem cells and started work toward developing them in the 1980s. He published an article in *Science* in

1984 reporting the culture of human blastocysts, the pre-implantation embryos from which stem cells are derived. But he discontinued the work because of the controversy it aroused in England.

(Extracted from https://www.nytimes.com)

Exercises

1. Read the article and write a possible title for it.

2. Answer the following questions according to the passage.

1) Why was Robert G. Edwards awarded the Nobel Prize?

2) What are the procedure of in vitro fertilization?

3) Why was in vitro fertilization not well accepted since the birth of the first tube baby?

4) What were the agreement between Dr. Edwards and Dr. Steptoe while practicing the in vitro fertilization?

5) What personalities had made Dr. Edwards successful?

UNIT 7 Neurology

Neurological disorders are medically defined as disorders that affect both the central and peripheral nerves. These disorders include epilepsy, Alzheimer disease and other dementias, cerebrovascular diseases, multiple sclerosis, Parkinson's disease, neuro-infections, brain tumors, traumatic disorders of the nervous system due to head trauma, and neurological disorders as a result of malnutrition.

Part I Intensive Reading

Alzheimer's Disease

Alzheimer's disease (AD), which was first described by German Bavarian psychiatrist and neurologist Alois Alzheimer in 1907, is the most common degenerative central nervous system disease in the elderly. It afflicts millions of older people worldwide, causing functional impairment, loss of time, reduced productivity, and immense economic hardship. It also results in great mental and emotional loss to the patient, caregivers, and society. While millions of dollars have been put into Alzheimer's research, its cause remains unclear.

Epidemiology

At present, there are 50 million AD patients worldwide. It is the single most common cause of dementia, comprising 70% of all cases. The majority of the patients with Alzheimer's have late-onset (around 65 years of age or later), while a few have early-onset during their 40s or 50s.

Geographical distribution of Alzheimer's is slightly skewed. The western European countries and North America have the highest prevalence of Alzheimer's, followed by China, Latin America, and Western-Pacific countries. The incidence rates also depict a similar picture, except for the fact that Latin America has a relatively higher incidence of Alzheimer's compared to the western European countries. The number of people with dementia is anticipated to double every 20 years. The age-specific prevalence of AD almost doubles every 5 years after aged 65. Among developed nations, approximately 1 in 10 older people (65+ years) is affected by some degree of dementia, whereas more than one third of very old people (85+ years) may have dementia-related symptoms and signs.

Mechanisms/Pathophysiology

- Etiological factors

    Aging. The most important risk factor in AD is aging. Younger individuals rarely have this disease, and most AD cases have a late onset that starts after 65 years of age.

    Genetics. Genetic factors were discovered over the years and were found to play a major role in the development of AD. About 70% of the AD cases were related to genetic factors.

- Pathogenesis

    AD is characterized by cognitive impairment, progressive neurodegeneration and formation of amyloid-β (Aβ)-containing plaques and neurofibrillary tangles composed of hyperphosphorylated tau. The neurodegenerative process in AD is initially characterized by synaptic damage accompanied by neuronal loss. In addition, recent evidence suggests that alterations in adult neurogenesis in the hippocampus might play a role. Synaptic loss is one of the strongest correlates to the cognitive impairment in patients with AD. Several lines of investigation support the notion that the synaptic pathology and defective neurogenesis in AD are related to progressive accumulation of Aβ oligomers rather than fibrils. Abnormal accumulation of Aβ resulting in the formation of toxic oligomers is the result of an imbalance between the levels of Aβ production, aggregation and clearance. Aβ oligomers might lead to synaptic damage by forming pore-like structures with channel activity; alterations in glutamate receptors; circuitry hyper-excitability; mitochondrial dysfunction; lysosomal failure and alterations in signaling pathways related to synaptic plasticity, neuronal cell and neurogenesis. A number of signaling proteins are involved in the neurodegenerative progression of AD. Therapies for AD might require the development of anti-aggregation compounds, pro-clearance pathways, and blockers of hyperactive signaling pathways.

Diagnosis

- Symptoms of AD

Many patients with Alzheimer's disease visit physicians at the request of concerned family members and are not brought in specifically for problems with cognition. It is therefore important to be alert for symptoms of possible dementia that may be evident clinically or in conversation with patients and family members. Signs of cognitive decline include memory loss affecting job performance, functioning, and social skills; mood and personality changes (e.g. apathy, depression, irritability); and difficulty with familiar tasks. The patients described in this section illustrate the importance of being alert to early warning signs of Alzheimer's disease, some of which may not overtly indicate memory loss.

- Diagnosis of AD

According to the National Alzheimer's Association, there is currently no single diagnostic test that can detect if a person has AD. However, new diagnostic tools and criteria make it possible for a physician to make a positive clinical diagnosis of AD with an accuracy of 85%-90%.

The diagnostic process generally takes more than one day and will involve the primary care physician and possibly other specialty physicians, such as a psychiatrist or neurologist. Here are the steps to diagnose Alzheimer's disease.

A complete medical history includes a patient's current mental or physical conditions, prescription drug intake, and family history of health problems.

A mental status evaluation assesses a person's sense of time and space, and his or her ability to remember, understand, talk, and do simple calculations. The person may be asked, "What year is it?" "Who is the president of the United States?" The person may also be asked to complete mental exercises, such as writing a sentence or spelling a word backwards.

A physical examination includes the evaluation of a person's nutritional status, blood pressure and pulse. These tests are done to rule out other potential causes of dementia, such as cardiac, respiratory, liver, kidney, or thyroid disease, and atherosclerosis.

A neurological examination tests the nervous system (brain and spinal cord) for evidence of other neurological disorders, such as stroke, Parkinson's disease, brain tumor or hydrocephalus (excess fluid in the brain), that may cause dementia-like symptoms. In this part of the examination physicians evaluate coordination, muscle tone and strength, eye movement, speech and sensory abilities.

Laboratory tests may be ordered to rule out other disorders that may be causing dementia. Blood and urine tests are used to check for anemia, infections, diabetes, kidney and liver disorders, nutritional deficiencies, and abnormally high or low levels of thyroid hormone. Brain imaging techniques, such as a CT scan or MRI, may be ordered to rule out the presence of tumors, stroke, blood clots, or other factors that may be causing memory and thinking problems. Genetic testing, with appropriate consents, can be used to identify autosomal dominant causes of AD where these are suspected. The increasing availability of genetic panels using next generation sequencing allows for large numbers of genes to be tested concurrently at reasonable costs.

Psychiatric, psychological and other evaluations are designed to rule out the presence of other illnesses such as depression, which might cause symptoms similar to those seen in AD. These evaluations test memory, reasoning, writing, vision-motor coordination, the ability to express ideas, and generally provide more in-depth information than the mental status evaluation alone.

There is no one or combination of diagnostic tests that will conclusively result in a diagnosis of AD. The tests will, however, help rule out other possible causes of the dementia-like symptoms. Once testing is completed, the diagnosing physician will review the results of the examinations, laboratory tests and other consultations to arrive at a diagnosis. If all test results appear to be consistent with Alzheimer's disease, the clinical diagnosis is generally "probable Alzheimer's disease", or "dementia of the Alzheimer type". If the symptoms are not typical, but no other cause is found, the diagnosis may be "possible Alzheimer's disease". A definitive diagnosis of AD can only be obtained upon autopsy of the brain at death.

Management

- Pharmacologic treatment

Given that there is presently no cure for Alzheimer's disease, the goal of treatment is to improve, stabilize, or slow the cognitive, functional, and behavioral decline. Pharmacologic treatments for Alzheimer's disease recommended by the American Academy of Neurology include the cholinesterase (ChE) inhibitors as a treatment standard and vitamin E as a treatment guideline. Although the role of this antioxidant in Alzheimer's disease is unclear, vitamin E has been shown to delay the time to clinical worsening in a double-blind trial.

Currently, the ChE inhibitors are the only U. S. Food and Drug Administration-approved drugs for the treatment of mild-to-moderate Alzheimer's disease. The widely accepted cholinergic hypothesis attributes the cognitive decline associated with

Alzheimer's disease in part to a loss of cholinergic neurons in the basal forebrain. By inhibiting enzymes that metabolize acetylcholine (ACh), ChE inhibitors increase ACh levels and thereby enhance cholinergic neurotransmission.

- Management of behavioral and neuropsychiatric disturbances

Alzheimer's disease patients commonly experience neuropsychiatric and behavioral disturbances such as agitation, depression, apathy and wandering. Physicians should probe the development of behavioral disturbances with the caregiver and patient, as attending to these disturbances is crucial to successful management of Alzheimer's disease. Generally, depressive symptoms manifest in early Alzheimer's disease while agitation, insomnia, fearfulness, and psychoses develop in moderate-to-severe stages. Behavioral symptoms may reemerge throughout the course of the disease.

Neuropsychiatric and behavioral disturbances are a particularly distressing aspect of Alzheimer's disease and are often the precipitant for nursing home placement. This is a significant issue for caregivers who prefer to have their loved ones at home for as long as possible. Importantly, slight improvements in behavior may facilitate patient manageability and delay placement into nursing facilities. Accordingly, family intervention programs and ChE inhibitor treatment have been demonstrated to keep patients at home longer.

Quality of Life

Prodromal and mild AD patients both suffered from worse QoL compared to a general population sample with similar demographic and clinical characteristics. Taking care of a family member with AD also exerts a lot of burden to the caregiver. There is strong support for exploiting the possibility of offering functional, emotional and financial support to the caregiver. The development and implementation of a National Action Plan on AD disease are of the utmost importance not only in terms of supporting patients and their caregivers but also in terms of achieving long-term rationalization of state resources available for the disease.

Prevention

Seven guidelines have emerged and are as follows:

1. Minimize your intake of saturated fats and trans fats. Saturated fat is found primarily in dairy products, meats, and certain oils (coconut and palm oils). Trans fats are found in many snack pastries and fried foods and are listed on labels as

"partially hydrogenated oils".

2. Vegetables, legumes (beans, peas, and lentils), fruits, and whole grains should replace meats and dairy products as primary staples of the diet.

3. Vitamin E should come from foods, rather than supplements. Healthful food sources of vitamin E include seeds, nuts, green leafy vegetables and whole grains. The recommended dietary allowance for vitamin E is 15 mg per day.

4. A reliable source of vitamin B12, such as fortified foods or a supplement providing at least the recommended daily allowance (2. 4 μg per day for adults), should be part of your daily diet. Have your blood levels of vitamin B12 checked regularly as many factors including age, may impair absorption.

5. If using multiple vitamins, choose those without iron and copper and consume iron supplements only when directed by your physician.

6. Although aluminum's role in Alzheimer's disease remains a matter of investigation, those who desire to minimize their exposure can avoid the use of cookware, antacids, baking powder, or other products that contain aluminum.

7. Include aerobic exercise in your routine, equivalent to 40 minutes of brisk walking 3 times per week.

(Extracted from https://pubmed. nobi. nlm. nih. gov)

Vocabulary

skewed	[skjuːd]	adj. 斜交的;歪斜的
amyloid	[ˈæmɪˌlɔɪd]	adj. 类淀粉的
neurofibrillary	[njʊərəˈfaɪbrɪleɪ]	n. 神经原纤维
hyperphosphorylated	[haɪpəfɒsfərɪˈleɪtɪd]	adj. 过度磷酸化的
tau	[tɔː]	n. 蛋白
synaptic	[sɪˈnæptɪk]	adj. 突触的
alteration	[ˌɔːltəˈreɪʃn]	n. 改变;变更
hippocampus	[ˌhɪpəˈkæmpəs]	n. 海马
oligomer	[əˈlɪgəmə]	n. 低聚体
fibril	[ˈfaɪbrɪl]	n. 纤维;原纤维
glutamate	[ˈgluːtəmeɪt]	n. 谷氨酸盐;谷氨酸酯
mitochondrial	[ˌmaɪtəʊˈkɒndrɪəl]	adj. 线粒体的
lysosomal	[ˌlaɪsəˈsəʊməl]	n. 溶酶体
aggregation	[ˌægrɪˈgeɪʃn]	n. 集合;聚合
apathy	[ˈæpəθɪ]	n. 冷漠
atherosclerosis	[ˌæθərəʊsklɪˈrəʊsɪs]	n. 动脉粥样硬化

hydrocephalus	[ˌhaɪdrəʊˈsefələs]	n. 脑水肿；脑积水
cholinesterase	[kəʊləˈnestəreɪs]	n. 胆碱酯酶
cholinergic	[ˌkəʊlɪˈnɜːdʒɪk]	adj. 胆碱（功）能的
acetylcholine	[ˌæsɪtɪlˈkɒliːn]	n. 乙酰胆碱
agitation	[ˌædʒɪˈteɪʃn]	n. 激动
neuropsychiatric	[njʊərəʊsaɪˈkɪætrɪk]	adj. 神经精神病学的
prodromal	[ˈprəʊdrəʊməl]	adj. 前驱症状的
hydrogenated	[haɪˈdrɒdʒəneɪtɪd]	adj. 氢化的
legume	[ˈlegjuːm]	n. 豆类；豆荚
fortified	[ˈfɔːtɪfaɪd]	adj. 加强的
aerobic	[eəˈrəʊbɪk]	adj. 有氧的

Exercises

1. Read the text and explain the following medical phrases.

1) Geographical distribution of AD

2) Pathological characters of AD

3) Symptoms of AD

4) Steps to diagnose AD

5) Goal of treating AD

2. Answer the following questions according to the text.

1) How does AD affect people?

2) What is the age range for AD patients?

3) What is the neurodegenerative process of AD?

4) What are the behavioral symptoms of AD?

3. Fill in the blanks with the proper forms of the given words.

> guarantee   mutate   presenilin   APP   Alzheimer
> implicate   onset   encode   unlike   individual

In a small percent of those diagnosed with 1)_____ disease the development of the disease can be attributed to genetic 2)_____. Three genes have been 3)_____ in its development. These are the genes which 4)_____ for amyloid precursor protein （APP）, the genes for presenilin-1 and for presenilin-2. Mutations in both the 5)_____ gene and the presenilin-1 gene result in 6)_____ development of the disease, while a mutation in the 7)_____-2 gene leads to a 95% chance of its development. 8)_____ with mutations in any of these three genes will usually develop symptoms as young as age 30, 9)_____ the vast majority of Alzheimer's cases, which are late 10)_____ where symptoms typically develop at age 65 and over.

4. **Study the bold-faced words in each of the following sentences and imitate the particular way of writing.**

Mentor Sentence:

☆ In morbidly obese patients, bariatric surgery **can be an effective means of** weight loss.

Imitation Sentence:

☆ Parenteral vaccination **can be an effective means of** inducing protective mucosal responses.

1) Alzheimer's disease, **which was first described by** German Bavarian psychiatrist and neurologist Alois Alzheimer in 1907, **is the most common** degenerative central nervous system disease in the elderly.

Answer: _____ **which was first described by** _____ **is the most common** _____

2) **Many patients with** Alzheimer's disease **visit physicians at the request of** concerned family members and are not brought in specifically for problems with cognition.

Answer: **Many patients with** _____ **visit physicians at the request of** _____

_____

3) **In this part of the exam, physicians evaluate** coordination, muscle tone and strength, eye movement, speech, and sensory abilities.

Answer: **In this part of the exam, physicians evaluate** _____

_____

4) Alzheimer's disease patients **commonly experience** neuropsychiatric and behavioral disturbances such as agitation, depression, apathy, and wandering.

Answer: _____ **commonly experience(s)** _____

_____

5. **Match the following statements with the corresponding sections in the text.**

Epidemiology:_____   Management:_____

Mechanisms/Pathophysiology: _____   Quality of Life:_____

Diagnosis:_____   Prevention:_____

A. Alzheimer's disease is an unavoidable neurological disorder in which the death of brain cells causes memory loss and cognitive decline and ultimate dementia.

B. It is the most common cause of dementia in people of 65 years and older.

C. It affects 10% of people over the age of 65 and 50% over the age of 85 years.

D. Approximately 4 million Alzheimer's patients are in the United States and the annual treatment costs are $100 billion.

E. It is the fourth leading cause of death in the United States and is becoming prevalent in many other countries.

F. The total brain size shrinks with Alzheimer's—the tissue has progressively fewer nerve cells and connections.

G. As such there is no known cure for Alzheimer's disease and the death of brain cells in the dementia cannot be halted or reversed.

H. Along with an aim to improve research into prevention and treatment, the goals of the plan also include measures for present interventions.

I. Help the people with Alzheimer's disease and their families, and enhance public awareness and engagement.

J. Enhance care quality and efficiency.

K. There are no disease-modifying drugs available for Alzheimer's disease but some options may reduce its symptoms and help improve quality of life and thereby help the patients to some extent.

L. There are four drugs in a class called cholinesterase inhibitor approved for symptomatic relief, i.e. donepezil, galantamine, rivastigmine and tacrine.

M. A different kind of drug, memantine (Namenda), an N-methyl-D-aspartate (NMDA) receptor antagonist, may also be used, alone or in combination with a cholinesterase inhibitor.

N. As with other types of dementia and neurodegenerative disease, a major part of therapy for patients with Alzheimer's comes from the support given by healthcare workers to provide dementia quality-of-life care, which becomes more important as needs increase with declining independence and increasing dependence.

6. Read the introduction in the box and finish the exercises after it.

> ***Top-down pattern*** *begins with the topic sentence followed by multiple levels of details and examples referred to as primary and secondary support. The primary support is more detailed and the secondary support is even more specific. These primary and secondary levels of support give concrete illustrations and provide credibility for the topic.*

1) Single-line the primary support and double-line the secondary support.

Dr. Alzheimer also found two types of deposits in Deter's brain. One kind was found outside the brain cells, which are known as plaques, and the other type of deposit was found inside brain cells, known as "neurofibrillary tangles". These plaques impair synapses so signals cannot pass between brain cells. Tangles kill brain cells by preventing the normal transport of food and energy around the brain cell.

2) Reorder the following sentences to make an effective paragraph.

A. The amount of time required for caregiving increases as dementia progresses; one study showed that people with dementia required 151 hours of caregiving per month at the outset of dementia and increased to 283 hours per month eight years later.

B. An analysis of national caregiving trends from 1999 to 2015 found that the average hours of care per week increased from 45 in 1999 to 48 in 2015 for dementia caregivers; over the same time period, weekly hours of care decreased for non-dementia caregivers from 34 to 24.

C. Apart from its long duration, caregiving for patients with Alzheimer's disease involves immediate demands that are also time-intensive.

D. Each instance of a decrease in an ADL or IADL in someone with dementia results in close to five more hours of monthly caregiving compared with a similar functional decrease for someone without dementia.

E. Caregivers of people with dementia report providing 27 hours more care per month on average (92 hours versus 65 hours) than caregivers of people without dementia.

Answer: __ __ __ __ __

7. Translate the Chinese paragraph below into English.

阿尔茨海默病是一种起病隐匿且进行性发展的神经系统退行性疾病。临床上以记忆障碍、失语、失用、失认、视空间技能损害、执行功能障碍及人格和行为改变等全面性痴呆表现为特征,病因迄今未明。

8. Read the text and fill in the sheet with proper information.

Reading Prompts	
Items	**Your Answers**
1) *Identify the medical terms concerning* **AD** *and group them according to your understanding.*	

continued

Reading Prompts	
Items	**Your Answers**
2) *Identify the* **adjectives** *used in* " **Epidemiology**" *and explain what conditions they describe.*	
3) *Identify the* **conjunctions** *used in* "**Diagnosis of AD**" *and point out the logical relation each of them indicates.*	
4) *Identify the* **verbs** *used in* **Exercise 3** *and point out the changes of verb tenses.*	
5) *Identify the* **typical sentence patterns.** (*the whole article*)	
6) *Identify the* **topic sentence** *and the* **supporting sentences** *in* "**Pathogenesis**".	

Title: _____

Dementia is an illness that affects the brain and eventually causes a person to lose the ability to perform daily self-care. All areas of daily living are affected over the course of the disease. Over time, a person with dementia loses the ability to learn new information, make decisions, and plan the future. Communication with other people becomes difficult. People with dementia ultimately lose the ability to perform daily tasks and to recognize the world around them.

In the beginning of the disease, the person may be aware of some changes in memory and rely more on others for reminders. As dementia worsens, the person may get lost easily and be unable to drive or manage finances. In advanced dementia, the person will lose the ability to eat, drink, bathe, dress, or use the toilet without assistance. Eventually, someone who is dying of dementia may not be able to swallow safely, talk, or get out of bed and will be totally dependent on others for help with every daily activity. Throughout the course of the disease, individuals may become sad or agitated, even wander or resist care. These behaviors are a form of communication that signifies the person's emotional condition and reactions to care.

Dementia also affects family caregivers

Seventy percent of persons with dementia live in the community, and family caregivers are largely responsible for helping them to remain at home. Family caregivers must be vigilant 24 hours a day to make sure that the person with dementia is safe and well. Their responsibilities include: housekeeping; shopping; managing finances; managing medications; helping with daily activities, such as eating, drinking, bathing, and dressing; ensuring that someone who wanders can do so safely; and overseeing other health care needs which may include conditions like diabetes or heart disease.

Providing constant, complicated care to a person with dementia takes a toll on family caregivers. Family members and other unpaid caregivers of people with Alzheimer's and other dementias are more likely than non-caregivers to report that their health is fair or poor.

Sources of stress to family caregivers

- Demographic stress

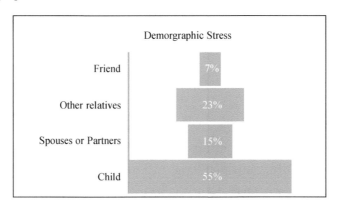

Figure 1　Caregiver demographics

Figure 1 illustrates caregiver demographics. Because of demographic changes in the U. S. population (i. e. parents of dependent minors are older than in the past and the U. S. population is aging), we now have something called the sandwich-generation caregiver, or a middle-aged person who simultaneously cares for dependent minor children and aging parents. The report found that 30% of AD and dementia caregivers had children under 18-year-old living with them and that 8%–13% of households in the United States had sandwich-generation caregivers. Such caregivers experience many challenges, such as limited time, energy, and financial resources, when balancing the care of both aging parents and dependent children. Because of these unique challenges, such caregivers may experience increased anxiety and depression and a decreased quality of life.

- Work-related stress

Family caregivers also experience work-related stress, such as the need to adjust their work schedule to accommodate caring for their loved one. About 57% of caregivers had to go in to work late, leave early, or take time off; that 16% had to take a leave of absence; and that 18% had to change from full-time to part-time work, a 5% increase in 2017 over 2016 data. Other work-related issues caregivers experienced were having to take a less demanding job, having to give up working entirely, receiving a warning about performance or attendance, and having to retire early.

- Time-related stress

Another stressful issue for families and caregivers is finding enough time to visit a loved one who is in a skilled care facility. If the loved one is cared for at home, the issue may be finding substitute caregivers when primary caregivers have other demands on their time. Issues may also arise with balancing the time needed to care for the patient with the time needed to care for self or other family members. Almost 23% of all caregivers are "on-duty" caregivers spending 24 hours a day, 7 day a week, caring for the loved one. Interestingly, 59% of those who were not on-duty caregivers felt as if they were. Women are 2.5 times more likely than men to provide on-duty care in the late stage of disease.

Caregiver intervention is an important area where more support is needed. If the health and wellbeing of caregivers are neglected, those they care for will suffer as well. The desired outcome of caregiver intervention is successful management of stress and depression, which in turn delays the need to admit the AD patient to a nursing home. Some examples of intervention include counseling, support groups, case management support, and respite care, all of which can help caregivers be their best for the patient.

- Physical and emotional stress

Reports from 2014 and 2018 cite both physical and emotional stress as being other burdens placed on families; 47% of women and 24% of men considered their caregiving role to be physically stressful, and 62% of women and 52% of men considered their caregiving role to be emotionally stressful. Adding to the stress is that 51% of caregivers have no medical experience, creating difficulty with making decisions or knowing what to do next.

(Extracted from *Journal of Nuclear Medicine Technology*)

Exercises

1. **Read the article and write a possible title for it.**

2. **Answer the following questions according to the passage.**

　　1) How does dementia influence patients?

　　2) What types of stress may caregivers of dementia experience?

　　3) What are the demographic features of caregivers for dementia?

　　4) What does "on-duty" caregivers have to confront with?

　　5) Do you have any good ideas on caring for dementia?

UNIT 8 Stomatology

Stomatology or dentistry is the branch of medicine concerned with the structures, functions, and diseases of the mouth. Tooth problems cover cavities, worn tooth enamel or fillings, gum disease, fractured teeth, and exposed roots. Patients might need fillings, root canals, or treatment of gums once a dentist diagnoses the problem.

Part I Intensive Reading

Dental Caries

Dental caries refers to the localized destruction of susceptible dental hard tissues by acidic by-products from the bacterial fermentation of dietary carbohydrates. It is a chronic disease that progresses slowly in most people, which results from an ecological imbalance in the equilibrium between tooth minerals and oral biofilms (plaque).

Epidemiology

Dental caries are the most important global oral health problem. Globally, it is estimated that 60%-90% of young people (children and adolescents) and 100% of the adult population experience dental caries. The disease is most prevalent in Latin American countries, countries in the Middle East, and South Asia, and least prevalent in China. In the United States, dental caries is the most common chronic childhood disease, being at least five times more common than asthma. It is the primary pathological cause of tooth loss in children. Between 29% and 59% of adults over the age of fifty experience caries.

Mechanisms/Pathophysiology

- Pathogenesis

The classic description of the cause of dental caries includes three factors: host, bacteria and diet. Dental caries occurs when a susceptible tooth surface is colonized with cariogenic bacteria and dietary source of sucrose or refined sugar is present. Bacterial pathogen produced lactic acid from fermentation of carbohydrates and this acid dissolves the hydroxyapatite crystal structure of the tooth, which causes caries.

Action mechanisms that lead to dental caries development

Dental caries is clinically characterized by a large polymorphism and a very complex etiology. Dental caries begins when there is a favorable interaction between multiple etiological factors that create an imbalance in the oral cavity which allows the development of the disease.

A carious lesion initiates with the production of organic acids by the microorganisms of the oral cavity, namely S. mutans and Lactobacillus, which metabolize the extracellular carbohydrates of the individual's diet. The presence of the organic acids will decrease the pH in the interface between the tooth surface and the bacterial plaque, allowing the development of the demineralization process on the tooth enamel. In the mouth, these changes over time are known as Stephan responses or Stephan curves. The pH of dental plaque under resting conditions (when no food or drink has been consumed) is fairly constant. The response after exposure of dental plaque to a fermentable carbohydrate is that pH decreases rapidly, reaching a minimum in approximately 5 to 20 minutes. This is followed by a gradual recovery to its starting value, usually over 30 to 60 minutes, although this can be longer in some individuals. When the oral cavity has a pH below 5.5 (considered as the critical pH), the saturation of the dental tissues initiates causing demineralization. If this process is frequent and constant, an initial lesion will initiate and it may become the precursor of a dental caries.

- Etiological factors of dental caries

Primary etiological factors

There are three main etiological factors that are essential for the initiation and development of the disease:

    □ *susceptible host*

    □ *cariogenic oral microflora*

□ *substrate that depends on the host's diet, which is then metabolized by the microorganisms that constitute that bacterial plaque*

Secondary etiological factors

□ *Time.* The time factor has an important role in the manifestation of clinical signs of the development of caries lesions. This factor was added to the primary etiological factors, since these need to be present for a certain period of time, so that the progressive demineralization of enamel may develop.

□ *Fluorides.* Fluoride is most effective in dental caries prevention when a low level of fluorides is constantly maintained in the oral cavity. It can be obtained from fluoridated drinking water, salt, milk, mouth rinse or toothpaste as well as professionally applied fluorides, or from combinations of fluoridated toothpaste with either of the other two fluoride sources.

□ *Saliva.* The oral cavity is constantly exposed to many different kinds of substances, some of which influence the caries process to a great extent. An important function of saliva is therefore the dilution and elimination of substances introduced into the oral cavity, through a physiological process usually referred to as salivary clearance or oral clearance. In patients with reduced quantity of saliva, the mechanistic and cleaning properties of this fluid in the mouth are impaired. With regard to prolonged oral clearance, a low oral sugar clearance inevitably increases the risk of caries development.

- Pathophysiology

Enamel

Demineralization of enamel by caries follows the direction of the enamel rods and the different triangular patterns between pit and fissure and smooth-surface caries develop in the enamel. As the enamel loses minerals, the enamel develops several distinct zones: translucent zone, dark zone, body of the lesion, and surface zone. The translucent zone coincides with $1\%-2\%$ loss of minerals. The dark zone is the slight remineralization of enamel. The greatest demineralization and destruction are in the body of the lesion. The surface zone remains relatively mineralized until the loss of tooth structure results in a cavitation.

Dentine

In dentine from the deepest layer to the enamel, the distinct areas affected by caries are the advancing front, the zone of bacterial penetration, and the zone of destruction. The advancing front represents a zone of demineralized dentine due to acid and has no bacteria present. The zones of bacterial penetration and destruction are the locations of invading bacteria and ultimately the decomposition of dentin. The zone of destruction has a more mixed bacterial population where proteolytic enzymes have destroyed the organic matrix.

Cementum

The incidence of cemental caries increases in older adults as gingival slump occurs from either trauma or periodontal disease. It is a chronic condition that forms a large, shallow lesion and slowly invades first the root's cementum and then dentin to cause a chronic infection of the pulp.

Diagnosis

Primary diagnosis. Initially it may appear as a small chalky area (smooth surface caries) which may eventually develop into a large cavitation. Inspection of all visible tooth surfaces is conducted by using a good light source, dental mirror and explorer. Dental radiographs (X-rays) are used for less visible areas of teeth in particular caries between the teeth. Lasers without ionizing radiation also now used for detection of interproximal decay (between the teeth). Visual and tactile inspection along with radiographs are employed frequently among dentists, in particular to diagnose pit and fissure caries. Early, uncavitated caries is often diagnosed by blowing air across the suspect surface, which removes moisture and changes the optical properties of the unmineralized enamel.

Differential diagnosis. Dental fluorosis and developmental defects of the tooth including hypomineralization of the tooth and hypoplasia of the tooth are used for dental caries.

Clinical presentation. The signs and symptoms of cavities vary, depending on their extent and location. When a cavity is just beginning, it may not have any symptoms at all. As the decay gets larger, it may cause signs and symptoms such as:

□ *toothache and mild to sharp pain when eating or drinking something sweet, hot or cold called tooth sensitivity*

□ *visible holes or pits in teeth*

□ *brown, black or white staining on any surface of a tooth*

□ *bad breath and foul tastes*

□ *fever, chills, abscess and trismus*

Management

The goal of treatment is to preserve tooth structures and prevent further destruction of the tooth. Most importantly, whether the carious lesion is cavitated or noncavitated dictates the management. Noncavitated lesions can be arrested and remineralization can occur with extensive changes to the diet, that is, reduction in frequency of refined sugars. It can be treated with non-operative method by tooth remineralization.

- Tooth remineralization

Tooth remineralization is a process in which minerals are returned to the molecular structure of the tooth itself. Destroyed tooth structure does not fully regenerate, although remineralization of very small carious lesions may occur if dental hygiene is kept at an optimal level such as by tooth brushing twice per day with fluoride toothpaste and flossing, and regular application of topical fluoride. Such management of a carious lesion is termed "non-operative treatment". In cavitated lesions, especially if dentin is involved, remineralization is much more difficult, and a dental restoration is usually indicated. Such management of a carious lesion is termed "operative treatment".

- Dental restoration

A dental restoration or dental filling is a process in which dental restorative material (including dental amalgam, composite resin, porcelain and gold) is used to restore the function, integrity and morphology of missing tooth structure. Composite resin and porcelain can be made to match the color of a patient's natural teeth and are more frequently used. Local anesthetics, nitrous oxide, or other prescription medications may be required in some cases to relieve pain during or following treatment or to relieve anxiety during treatment.

- Tooth extraction

The removal of the decayed tooth is performed if the tooth is too far destroyed from the decay process to effectively restore the tooth.

- Dental sealants

A sealant is a thin plastic-like coating applied to the chewing surfaces of the molars to prevent food from being trapped inside pits and fissures.

Quality of Life

Dental caries is not only a problem in childhood but also occurs at a relatively constant rate throughout life. Oral conditions pertain to problems with eating, nutrition, interaction, and emotional and psychological functions, as well as the condition like discomfort, disability and oral impairment. Thus, tooth decay can exert a negative impact on activities of daily living and, consequently, quality of life. Incremental tooth loss is an important contributor to poor QoL. In dentistry, oral health care is no longer merely seen as the clinical appearance of oral health conditions or the treatment of diseases. More attention has been given to how effective dental treatment can improve different aspects of patients' lives.

Prevention

- Oral hygiene

Personal hygiene care consists of proper brushing and flossing daily. Proper brushing and flossing is to remove and prevent the formation of plaque or dental biofilm. Professional hygiene care consists of regular dental examinations and professional prophylaxis (cleaning).

- Dietary modification

Minimizing snacking is recommended, since snacking creates a continuous supply of nutrition for acid-creating bacteria in the mouth. Chewy and sticky foods (such as dried fruit or candy) tend to adhere to teeth longer, so brushing the teeth after meals is recommended. For children, the ADA and the EAPD recommend limiting the frequency of consumption of drinks with sugar, and not giving baby bottles to infants during sleep. Chewing gum containing xylitol (a sugar alcohol) helps in reducing dental biofilm.

- Calcium and fluoride

Calcium is found in food such as milk and green vegetables and is often recommended to protect against dental caries. Fluoride helps prevent decay of a tooth by binding to the hydroxyapatite crystals in enamel. The incorporated calcium makes enamel more resistant to demineralization, and thus resistant to decay. Topical fluoride includes a fluoride toothpaste, mouthwash or varnish is now more highly recommended than systemic intake such as by tablets or drops to protect the surface of the teeth. After brushing with fluoride toothpaste, rinsing should be avoided. Fluoride has pre-eruptive and post-eruptive effects on caries prevention.

(Extracted from https://www.researchgate.net)

Vocabulary

fermentation	[ˌfɜːrmenˈteɪʃn]	n. 发酵
biofilm	[ˌbaɪəufɪlm]	n. 生物膜
cariogenic	[ˌkeərɪəuˈdʒenɪk]	adj. 生龋齿的
sucrose	[ˈsuːkrəuz]	n. 蔗糖
lactic	[ˈlæktɪk]	adj. 乳汁的
hydroxyapatite	[haɪdrɒksɪˈæpətaɪt]	n. 羟磷灰石
polymorphism	[ˌpɒlɪˈmɔːfɪzəm]	n. 多型现象；多态性
demineralization	[deminərəlaɪˈzeɪʃn]	n. 脱盐；脱矿质作用

enamel	[ɪ'næml]	*n.* 珐琅质;釉质
dilution	[daɪ'luːʃn]	*n.* 稀释物;冲淡物
translucent	[trænz'luːsənt]	*adj.* 半透明的
dentine	['dentiːn]	*n.* 牙质;牙本质;齿质
proteolytic	[ˌprəʊtɪə'lɪtɪk]	*adj.* 蛋白质分解的
cementum	[sɪ'mentəm]	*n.* 牙骨质
interproximal	[ˌɪntə'prɒksɪməl]	*adj.* 邻间的
		n. 牙间齐整器
hypoplasia	[ˌhaɪpə'pleɪʒə]	*n.* 发育不全
porcelain	['pɔːsəlɪn]	*n.* 瓷;瓷器

Exercises

1. Read the text and explain the following medical phrases.

1) Clinical characteristics of dental caries

2) Risk factors for dental caries

3) Pathological features of dental caries

4) Signs and symptoms of dental caries

2. Answer the following questions according to the text.

1) What can cause dental caries?

2) How does a dentist diagnose dental caries?

3) How does a dentist diagnose pit and fissure caries?

4) What is the goal of treating dental caries?

3. Fill in the blanks with the proper forms of the given words.

life-threatening	oral	S. mutans	microbial	hygiene
grow	biofilm	fermentation	dental	infection

Dental caries, a chronic disease is unique among human and is one of the most common important global oral health problems in the world today. It is the destruction of dental hard acellular tissue by acidic by-products from the bacterial 1)_____ of dietary carbohydrates especially sucrose. It progresses slowly in most people which results from an ecological imbalance in the equilibrium between tooth minerals and oral 2)_____ which is characterized by microbial activity, resulting in fluctuations in plaque pH due to bacterial acid production, buffering action from saliva and the surrounding tooth structure. The 3)_____ community of caries is diverse and contains many facultatively and obligatelyanaerobic bacteria. 4)_____ is the most primary one associated with it. Dental caries can affect the patients in various ways, i. e. presence of tooth pain, 5)_____ or dysfunction of the stomatognathic system can limit the necessary ingestion of energetic foods, affecting the 6)_____ in children and adults as well as their learning, communication skills and recreational activities. Moreover, 7)_____ and pharyngeal cancers and oral tissue lesions are also a significant health concern. Cavernous sinus thrombosis and Ludwig's angina can be 8)_____. Due to this, treatment is needed for 9)_____ diseases and the cost is normally high and is not feasible for all of the community due to limited resources such as time, person and money. Therefore, prevention is more affordable. Personal 10)_____ care and dietary modification should be recommended.

4. **Study the bold-faced words in each of the following sentences and imitate the particular way of writing.**

Mentor Sentence:

☆ In morbidly obese patients, bariatric surgery **can be an effective means of** weight loss.

Imitation Sentence:

☆ Parenteral vaccination **can be an effective means of** inducing protective mucosal responses.

1) Dental caries **refers to** the localized destruction of susceptible dental hard tissues by acidic by-products from the bacterial fermentation of dietary carbohydrates.

Answer: _____ **refers to** _____

_____

2) Dental caries **is clinically characterized by** a large polymorphism and a very complex etiology.

Answer: _____ **is/are clinically characterized by** _____

_____

3) **With regard to** prolonged oral clearance, a low oral sugar clearance inevitably increases the risk of caries development.

Answer: **With regard to** _____

_____

4) Initially it may appear as a small chalky area (smooth surface caries) which **may eventually develop into** a large cavitation.

Answer: _____

_____ **may eventually develop into** _____

5. Match the following statements with the corresponding sections in the text.

Epidemiology:＿＿＿＿＿＿＿＿＿＿   Management:＿＿＿＿＿＿＿＿＿＿

Mechanisms/Pathophysiology:＿＿＿＿＿＿＿＿＿＿   Quality of Life:＿＿＿＿＿＿＿＿＿＿

Diagnosis:＿＿＿＿＿＿＿＿＿＿   Prevention:＿＿＿＿＿＿＿＿＿＿

A. The seriousness and societal costs of dental caries in preschool children are enormous.

B. National data shows that caries is highly prevalent in poor and near poor US preschool children, yet this disease is infrequently treated.

C. The etiology includes elevated colonization levels of mutans streptococci, high frequency sugar consumption, and developmental defects on primary teeth.

D. A necessary first step in preventing dental caries in preschool children is evaluating the child's caries risk factors which include socioeconomic status, previous carious experience, presence of white spot lesions, presence of visible plaque, perceived risk by dental professionals, and microbiologic testing for the presence or quantity of mutans streptococci.

E. Based on this knowledge, different preventive strategies as well as different intensities of preventive therapies can be employed.

F. Caries preventive strategies in preschool children include diet modifications to reduce high frequency sugar consumption, supervised tooth brushing with fluoridated dentifrice, systemic fluoride supplements to children living in a nonfluoridated area that are at risk for caries, professional topical fluoride with fluoride varnish, and sealants for primary molar.

6. Read the introduction in the box and finish the exercises after it.

> *Sometimes your core ideas are too new, complex, or jargon laden for a reader to follow in the top-down pattern. Good writers address this challenge by using a* **bottom-up** *paragraph structure, especially in the first paragraphs of a section. The paragraph begins with something (the beginning point) that every reader can relate to, then builds in complexity, and finally culminates in a new complex idea (the ending point).*

1) Single-line the beginning point and double-line the ending point.

The first step of plaque formation occurs when you break down food into carbohydrates while chewing. The carbohydrates then combine with the natural bacteria in your mouth to create an acid. This acid by itself is problematic because it can eat away at enamel. However, when the acid combines with left-behind particles of food and saliva, another chemical reaction occurs and the substance becomes sticky and somewhat hard. This new substance formed is plaque, and it sticks to your teeth, causing all sorts of problems if not removed.

2) Reorder the following sentences to make an effective paragraph.

A. So, it is important to take care of your teeth.

B. Healthy teeth help you speak clearly and allow you to eat a variety of foods, thereby helping you maintain a healthy diet.

C. Your teeth are more than just part of a beautiful smile.

D. A large national study found that people older than 65 years who had good dental health tended to be healthier overall.

Answer: ___ ___ ___ ___

7. Translate the Chinese paragraph below into English.

龋病是一种主要由细菌引起的慢性感染性疾病,是口腔内多种微生物共同作用的结果。龋病已成为很多口腔及全身疾病的直接或间接原因。龋病是口腔中的常见疾病,虽然病程发展较为缓慢,但是它发病率高且流行区域广泛。

8. Read the text and fill in the sheet with proper information.

Reading Prompts	
Items	**Your Answers**
1) *Identify the medical terms concerning **dental caries** and group them according to your understanding.*	
2) *Identify the **adjectives** used in "**Clinical presentation**" and explain what conditions they describe.*	
3) *Identify the **conjunctions** used in "**Quality of Life**" and point out the logical relation each of them indicates.*	

continued

Reading Prompts	
Items	**Your Answers**
4) *Identify the* **verbs** *used in* **Exercise 3** *and point out the changes of verb tenses.*	
5) *Identify the* **typical sentence patterns.** （**the whole article**）	
6) *Identify the* **topic sentence** *and the* **supporting sentences** *in* "**Dental restoration**".	

Title: _____

Until very recently, "false" teeth were often not false at all, but rather real teeth taken from another human or animal. The earliest record of dentures is from around 7th century BCE, when Etruscans fashioned dentures from animal and human teeth. This art ended with their civilization, but re-emerged with the practice of making dentures in the 1700s.

In the 1700s, sugar was well known and available throughout Europe. As a result, there was more tooth decay and tooth-saving techniques such as root canals were not yet developed. This meant that many people were missing teeth, and it was rare for someone to reach 50 with all their natural teeth. And so many people needed false teeth.

Early Types of False Teeth

Although our modern technology allows for comfort and easy-to-use dentures, this was not always the case. Original dentures had difficulties with fit, attachment, comfort and durability. As dentists tried to improve false teeth, they tried many different materials and techniques.

• Ivory

Ivory was one of the earliest materials used to replace lost teeth. Ivory came from animals like the hippopotamus, walrus or elephant. These teeth tended to decay and rarely looked natural, but got the job done. Ivory was still used for the base of dentures, even after quality human teeth became more available near the end of the 18th century.

• Waterloo Teeth

The best dentures were made from human teeth. The source of these teeth ranged from robbed graves, peasants looking to make a quick buck, and even dentists' collections. Understandably, these sources provided poor quality teeth. Their poor quality meant that dentures were mostly cosmetic and needed to be removed for eating.

The death of 50,000 men at the battle of Waterloo in 1815 soon diminished the lack of quality human teeth. Soldiers marching at Waterloo were young and healthy, so their teeth were ideal for denture making. "Waterloo teeth" became the fashion in Britain and were often worn as a trophy despite the impossibility of knowing their direct origin.

This practice of using human teeth for dentures continued into the late 1860s. The American Civil War provided one source to these later versions of "Waterloo teeth".

• Vulcanite

Luckily, such ghastly techniques lessened after 1843 when Charles Goodyear discovered how to make flexible rubber. Charles's brother Nelson named the new material vulcanite and patented it in 1851. It turns out that vulcanite makes a more comfortable base for false teeth. Because other versions of false teeth were more expensive, the market for vulcanite teeth flourished. For the first time ever, middle class people bought and wore false teeth along with the rich and wealthy.

• Porcelain

Porcelain false teeth were invented in the late 1700s in France. However, their tendency to crack and grate against each other made them unpopular choices. It wasn't until after many improvements in strength and texture in the late 1800s that porcelain teeth became a popular choice for dentures and bridges and replaced human teeth, ivory and bone. Porcelain is still a popular choice for many dental applications.

Famous Figures

Until recently, the wealthy were the only ones who could afford false teeth. Here are some wealthy public figures whose dental history you may find interesting.

• Queen Elizabeth I

In the time before common cavity prevention practices existed, problem teeth were extracted right and left. Few attempted replacements with substitute teeth, and the procedures often went awry. If aching teeth remained, further decay would occur with no replacement alternative.

During her 44 year reign from 1558 – 1603, ivory dentures had not yet been developed. As a result, the only solution available to her was stuffing bits of cloth into the gaps in her teeth when attending public events.

• George Washington

Even the great leaders can't be perfect. In George Washington's case, one big shortcoming was his infamously terrible teeth. Equally infamous, Washington's wooden dentures have become the stuff of legend, a factually incorrect legend, as Washington never actually sported dentures made from wood. Instead, Washington commissioned several dentists throughout his life to fashion false teeth out of the finest materials available. In his twenties, George began to lose teeth to decay and suffered from toothaches constantly over the years.

Before the Revolutionary War, Dr. John Baker made a partial denture of ivory to wire to Washington's remaining teeth. Later, Dr. John Greenwood of New York fashioned an advanced denture out of hippopotamus ivory for the president's inauguration in 1789. Dr. Greenwood even made a hole in the dentures for Washington's final remaining tooth, which Washington later gave to him as a thank you.

Modern Dentures

Luckily, for us, the 20th century yielded new technologies and materials for dentures. Acrylic resins and other moldable plastics are now the norm for denture and bridge partials. Plastics are easy to get and manipulate, so the price of dentures is also considerably lower.

Dental advancements also came about regarding the fit and suction of false teeth. Modern false teeth and dentures are more comfortable, are easier to chew with (yes, even corn on the cob), and last longer than teeth made with past materials. Although, far less people need false teeth and dentures now, thanks to advances in dental hygiene and dentistry.

(Extracted from https://silveradofamilydental.com)

Exercises

1. Read the article and write a possible title for it.

2. Answer the following questions according to the passage.

1) When did the earliest dentures appear?
2) Why were dentures urgently needed in Europe in the 1700s?
3) What materials had been used to make dentures in earlier time?
4) What materials are now used to make dentures?
5) What type of unhealthy habits may cause tooth problems?

UNIT 9 Pediatrics

Pediatrics is the branch of medicine for the health and medical care of infants, children and adolescents. Pediatric illnesses include colds, allergies, skin problems, eye conditions, neurological issues and gastrointestinal conditions etc. It's important to understand how different conditions affect certain age groups as well as the degree of severity.

Part I Intensive Reading

Neonatal Jaundice

Jaundice is the most common condition that requires medical attention and hospital readmission in newborns. The yellow coloration of the skin and sclera in newborns with jaundice is the result of accumulation of unconjugated bilirubin. In most infants, unconjugated hyperbilirubinemia reflects a normal transitional phenomenon. However, in some infants, serum bilirubin levels may rise excessively, which can be cause for concern because unconjugated bilirubin is neurotoxic and can cause death in newborns and lifelong neurologic sequelae in infants who survive kernicterus.

Epidemiology

The degree of neonatal jaundice in the healthy newborn infant has been shown to depend on many factors, including maternal race and parity, maternal diseases, gestational age, male sex, instrumental delivery, bruising, previous sibling with history of neonatal jaundice, weight loss, and breast-feeding. The relative importance of such influences on the occurrence of neonatal jaundice may vary in different populations. For example, the prevalence of high parity, teenage pregnancy, or maternal diseases in a population may be important for establishing norms for serum bilirubin levels.

Mechanism/Pathophysiology

Jaundice reflects the accumulation of the yellow-orange pigment bilirubin in the skin, sclera and other tissues; it does not imply any particular causation. Thus, preventive and therapeutic approaches to pathophysiologic neonatal jaundice or hyperbilirubinemia have typically been nonspecific. More specific or targeted approaches require a better understanding of the pathophysiology involved in each individual case.

The production of bilirubin as a result of the degradation of heme arising from normal red blood cell turnover is a normal part of our physiology. Bilirubin is normally conjugated and then excreted via the liver. It is transported in the bloodstream bound to albumin. Once entering hepatocytes, it is conjugated with glucuronic acid to form bilirubin glucuronide, also known as either "conjugated" or "direct" bilirubin.

Determining whether the hyperbilirubinemia is conjugated or unconjugated can reveal where bilirubin metabolism/clearance is defective and therefore give clues to the underlying etiology. Unconjugated hyperbilirubinemia can result from overproduction of bilirubin, impaired hepatic uptake, or abnormalities of bilirubin conjugation. Conjugated hyperbilirubinemia may be due to hepatocellular injury, intrahepatic cholestasis or biliary obstruction.

Newborn infants, particularly premature ones, have an immature bilirubin conjugation and excretion system. Neonatal jaundice reflects an increase in total body bilirubin load after birth, but the apparent or "visible" jaundice is not a good predictor of the level of bilirubin in circulation or the amount of bilirubin in the various tissues. As bilirubin can have toxic effects under some conditions, its levels need to be closely monitored in the first weeks after birth.

Diagnosis

Defining the severity of jaundice. The terms "physiological jaundice" and "pathological jaundice" lead to confusion and are best avoided. "Hyperbilirubinemia" is the simplest term to denote a raised level of bilirubin in the blood. "Clinical jaundice" is used to describe visually detectable jaundice, and "significant hyperbilirubinemia" to distinguish a level of jaundice requiring treatment.

Jaundice with a pathological cause. Clinical features that suggest a pathological cause of jaundice and prompt further investigation are as follows:

□ *jaundice appearing in the first 24 hours of life*

□ *jaundice in a sick neonate*

□ *rapidly rising serum bilirubin*

□ *prolonged jaundice more than 14 days in term infants; more than 21 days in preterm infants*

□ *conjugated serum bilirubin more than 25 μmol/liter*

□ *pale, chalky stools and dark urine*

Early-onset jaundice. Jaundice within the first 24 hours of life is likely to be the result of significant hemolysis. This is a neonatal emergency and a serum bilirubin measurement should be obtained within 2 hours. An urgent medical review should be conducted to establish the diagnosis. In the absence of hemolysis, rarer conditions affecting hepatic conjugation should be considered. Maternal blood group and rhesus status should be checked. Despite an ABO incompatibility set-up in 10%–15% of pregnancies, the number of cases that result in significant hemolysis is small. Other blood group incompatibilities will usually be known from the maternal history. The Kell group can cause severe hemolytic disease of the newborn.

The differential diagnosis of unconjugated jaundice. Details of gestational age and evidence of birth asphyxia and trauma may explain heightened or prolonged jaundice. The mode and success of feeding should be noted and assessment should be made of the infant's state of hydration and weight trend since birth. Examination of the newborn should be directed to signs of polycythemia, anemia, hydrops, purpura and frank bruising, along with features of infection. The maternal records should be checked for any history suggesting congenital infection and for documentation of syphilis and hepatitis serology.

The jaundice associated with galactosemia is likely to be predominantly unconjugated in the first week of life. Diagnostic pointers such as hepatomegaly, poor feeding and vomiting should prompt early screening for galactosemia with urinalysis for non-glucose reducing substances and assessment of erythrocyte galactose-1-phosphate uridyl transferase activity. With parents of Mediterranean, Asian and African ethnicity, the increased likelihood of G6PD (glucose-6-phosphate dehydrogenase) deficiency, especially in males, needs to be considered. G6PD levels can be falsely elevated in the context of a high reticulocyte count and so may need to be repeated at 2–3 months of age.

Prolonged jaundice. Visibly detectable jaundice beyond 2 weeks of age in the term infant and 3 weeks in the preterm is classified as "prolonged jaundice". The majority of term infants presenting with prolonged jaundice have an unconjugated hyperbilirubinemia and will be breastfeeding. Providing there are no features in the history or on clinical examination that suggest a pathological cause (in particular, the urine is not dark, stool color is not pale and chalky, or there is no hepatomegaly and the baby is thriving), screening investigations can be delayed until 3 weeks of age in the term infant. The total and conjugated serum bilirubin must be determined. Some of the following tests may be appropriate:

- □ *full blood count*
- □ *examination of blood film if hemolysis is suspected*
- □ *blood group and DAT (mother's group and antibody status should be known)*
- □ *thyroid function tests if result of heel-prick TSH screen is not known*
- □ *urinalysis for reducing sugars*
- □ *urinalysis for evidence of infection*

Cholestatic or conjugated jaundice. The definition of conjugated hyperbilirubinemia usually refers to a serum level more than 25 μmol/liter. Pale chalky stools and dark bile-stained urine are the clinical markers of established conjugated jaundice, but they may be absent in the first weeks of hepatic pathologies, including biliary atresia.

Diagnosis of any associated clotting abnormality and its correction are urgent considerations in the infant with conjugated jaundice. Several conditions present with a mixture of raised unconjugated and conjugated bilirubin. Notable amongst these are the intrauterine infections, bacterial sepsis, galactosemia, aminoacidemia and congenital hypopituitarism.

Management

Management of neonatal jaundice starts with prevention. The accepted treatments for unconjugated jaundice are phototherapy, exchange transfusion and high-dose intravenous immunoglobulin (IVIG) used to suppress isoimmune hemolysis.

Phototherapy. Phototherapy remains the most convenient and safe means of lowering serum bilirubin. Most importantly, phototherapy reduces the need for the more hazardous alternative, namely exchange transfusion. Phototherapy would only appear to be effective as bilirubin enters the skin at serum levels more than 80 μmol/liter. The maximal effects of phototherapy is during the first 24 − 48 hours of its use.

Phototherapy has a benign reputation but it is not without side effects. The more commonly encountered are:

□ *diarrhea*

□ *increased fluid loss via the skin*

□ *temperature instability*

□ *erythematous rashes*

□ *tanning*

□ *bronze baby syndrome*

Diarrhea and increased insensible water loss require attention to fluid balance. Close attention to thermoregulation is also important. The eyes of an infant receiving lamp phototherapy should be shielded to prevent potential retinal damage. The bronze baby syndrome results from an interaction between cholestatic jaundice and phototherapy. The brown pigment produced (bilifuscin) stains the infant's skin and lingers for some weeks after phototherapy has been discontinued.

Pharmacological agents. Administration of high-dose intravenous immunoglobulin (IVIG) has entered practice for newborns presenting with severe rhesus or ABO isoimmunization. Treatment significantly reduces the need for exchange transfusion, the duration of phototherapy and the length of hospital stay, but recipients are more likely to require top-up red cell transfusions for late anemia. As a precaution against over use of a pooled human blood product, it is recommended that IVIG be reserved for hemolyzing babies with a serum bilirubin that continues to climb at a rate more than 8.5 μmol/liter/h despite multiple phototherapy. The majority of cases of ABO incompatibility are amenable to multiple phototherapy if delivered optimally. A more pre-emptive use of IVIG may be called for in cases of severe rhesus disease where there has been little or no in utero management, or cases of ABO incompatibility readmitted with a serum bilirubin level approaching or above exchange values.

Exchange transfusion. Exchange transfusion will remain necessary for infants who fail to respond to optimal phototherapy or who present late with bilirubin levels in excess of a given exchange value. In the latter case, the infant should be placed under multiple phototherapy, and cross-matched blood should be sought as a matter of urgency for an anticipated exchange transfusion. Signs and symptoms of acute bilirubin encephalopathy are an absolute indication to proceed with an exchange transfusion. This may be informed by the peak serum bilirubin, the duration of jaundice, the bilirubin/albumin ratio and the clinical status of the baby.

Quality of Life

As virtually all neonates have decreased conjugation and excretion capabilities at birth, hyperbilirubinemia in the first 1 – 3 days of life almost always reflects an increase in bilirubin production. Jaundice presenting from days 3 – 7 more often reflects more modest increases in production. When combined with even modest increases in production, the consequences can be devastating, with a dramatic and rapid rise in bilirubin levels. Infants with decreased food intake, and thus decreased stooling, may also present with increased jaundice at this time, because of the increased re-uptake of excreted bilirubin by the intestines. This is seen with so-called breastfeeding failure jaundice, when an infant's milk intake is too low. Jaundice presenting after the first week of life rarely represents increased bilirubin production, but rather implies decreased excretory ability. This is when problems with liver disease and biliary obstructions tend to present. Failure to recognize this transition represents a serious clinical error: once jaundice persists beyond 7 – 10 days, and certainly beyond 14 days, conjugated hyperbilirubinemia must be considered and ruled out to avoid delaying the diagnosis of biliary atresia.

Prevention

A clinical review within 48 hours of birth of babies has the following risk factors for significant hyperbilirubinemia:

　□ *gestational age under 38 weeks*
　□ *a previous sibling with neonatal jaundice requiring phototherapy*
　□ *mother's intention to breastfeed exclusively*
　□ *visible jaundice in the first 24 hours of life*

Clinical jaundice is more difficult to recognize in babies with dark skin tones and can be missed without close examination of the sclera, gums and blanched skin. These babies fall into the heightened risk group if they are not examined properly. In cases of doubt, a low threshold should be adopted for checking the transcutaneous or serum bilirubin.

(Extracted from https://www.pediatr-neonatol.com)

Vocabulary

neonatal	[ˌniːəʊˈneɪtl]	*adj*. 新生的；初生的
jaundice	[ˈdʒɔːndɪs]	*n*. 黄疸
hyperbilirubinemia	[haɪpɜːbiliːrʌbaɪˈniːmɪə]	*n*. 高胆红素血；血胆红素过多
sequela	[sɪˈkwiːlə]	*n*. 后遗症；并发症
hydration	[haɪˈdreɪʃn]	*n*. 水合作用
polycythemia	[ˌpɒlɪsaɪˈθiːmjə]	*n*. 红血球增多症
hydrops	[ˈhaɪdrɒps]	*n*. 积水
purpura	[ˈpɜːpjʊrə]	*n*. 紫癜

bruising	['bruːzɪŋ]	n. 挫伤的
syphilis	['sɪfɪlɪs]	n. 梅毒
serology	[sɪə'rɒlədʒɪ]	n. 血清学
galactosemia	[gəlæktə'siːmɪə]	n. 半乳糖血症
hepatomegaly	[hepətəʊ'megəlɪ]	n. 肝肿大
urinalysis	[ˌjʊərɪ'nælɪsɪs]	n. 验尿
reticulocyte	[rɪ'tɪkjʊləsaɪt]	n. 网状细胞
cholestatic	[kɒls'tətɪk]	adj. 胆汁阻塞的;胆汁郁积的
biliary atresia		胆管闭锁
aminoacidemia	[æmɪnəʊ'saɪdiːmɪə]	n. 氨基酸血症
sepsis	['sepsɪs]	n. 败血症
hypopituitarism	[ˌhaɪpəʊpɪ'tjuːɪtəˌrɪzəm]	n. 垂体机能减退
immunoglobulin	[ˌɪmjʊnəʊ'glɒbjʊlɪn]	n. 免疫球蛋白
bilifuscin	[bɪlɪ'fʊsɪn]	n. 胆褐素
isoimmunization	[aɪsəʊɪmjʊnaɪ'zeɪʃn]	n. 同种免疫
encephalopathy	[enˌsefə'lɒpəθɪ]	n. 脑病
transcutaneous	[ˌtrænzkjʊ'teɪnɪəs]	adj. 经皮的

Exercises

1. Read the text and explain the following medical phrases.

1) Definition of neonatal jaundice

2) Differences between unconjugated and conjugated hyperbilirubinemia

3) Diagnosis of neonatal jaundice

4) Treatment of neonatal jaundice

5) Side effects of phototherapy

2. Answer the following questions according to the text.

1) Which term can concisely denote jaundice?

2) What are the clinical features of neonatal jaundice?

3) What are the side effects of phototherapy on treating jaundice?

4) What risk factors should be noticed while preventing hyperbilirubinemia?

3. Fill in the blanks with the proper forms of the given words.

| physiology | breastfeed | type | pediatric | blue |
| formula-fed | bilirubin | premature | hydrate | white |

Most newborns have some jaundice, often called " 1) _____ " or "normal" jaundice, in the first week or so after birth. Just after birth, there is often extra 2)_____ from the breakdown of red blood cells, and the baby's liver is still developing, so this can lead to extra bilirubin in the blood for a short period of time. In 3)_____ babies, jaundice often lasts for 3 weeks or more. In 4)_____ babies, most jaundice goes away by 2 weeks.

Jaundice is more common in babies who are breastfed, particularly babies who are having difficulty nursing. Jaundice is also more common in babies who are 5)_____. In some cases, jaundice can be due to the baby having a different blood 6)_____ than the mother, often called "blood type incompatibility".

The best way to view your baby's skin is in good light, such as natural sunlight or bright fluorescent lights. Jaundice usually appears first in the face. As the amount of bilirubin in the blood increases, bilirubin can be seen in lower parts of the body such as the chest, then abdomen, and then legs. The 7)_____ of the eyes may also appear yellow.

Many babies have jaundice and most do not have problems or need treatment. If the level of bilirubin gets very high, it can possibly cause damage to the hearing and brain.

Your 8)_____ can test the level of bilirubin in your baby's blood to see if treatment is needed. Most babies with jaundice do not need treatment and the jaundice goes away on its own.

If you are breastfeeding, you should nurse your baby at least 8 to 12 times a day for the first few days. This will produce enough milk to keep your baby 9)_____ and help keep the bilirubin level low. If you are having trouble breastfeeding, talk with your baby's doctor about whether a lactation specialist can help. If treatment for jaundice is needed, that treatment often involves placing your baby under special 10)_____ lights called "bilirubin lights" or "bili lights". These lights help the bilirubin in the skin to break down and thereby lower the amount in the blood.

4. Study the bold-faced words in each of the following sentences and imitate the particular way of writing.

Mentor Sentence:

☆ In morbidly obese patients, bariatric surgery **can be an effective means of** weight loss.

Imitation Sentence:

☆ Parenteral vaccination **can be an effective means of** inducing protective mucosal responses.

1) The production of bilirubin **as a result of** the degradation of heme arising from normal red blood cell turnover is a normal part of our physiology.

Answer: _____ **as a result of** _____

_____

2) Jaundice within the first 24 hours of life **is likely to be** the result of significant hemolysis.

Answer: _____ **is/are likely to be** _____

_____

3) **In the absence of** hemolysis, rarer conditions affecting hepatic conjugation **should be considered.**

Answer: **In the absence of** _____

_____ **should be considered.**

4) Other blood group incompatibilities will usually be **known from** the maternal history.

Answer: _____ **known from**

5. **Match the following statements with the corresponding sections in the text.**

Epidemiology: _____   Management: _____

Mechanisms/Pathophysiology: _____   Quality of Life: _____

Diagnosis: _____   Prevention: _____

A. In cases of isoimmune hemolysis, high-dose immunoglobulin is indicated if the serum bilirubin is continuing to rise despite multiple phototherapy.

B. Jaundice is the most common clinical sign in neonatal medicine.

C. It can result from increased bilirubin production, inability of the liver to conjugate bilirubin or failure to excrete bilirubin into the biliary tree.

D. Phototherapy remains the mainstay of treatment of significant unconjugated hyperbilirubinemia, and its optimal use should keep the level of jaundice below the threshold for exchange blood transfusion.

E. The importance of identifying conjugated hyperbilirubinemia at an early stage cannot be overstated.

F. For babies with prolonged jaundice, investigation should be directed towards making a timely diagnosis and avoiding secondary complications.

G. Appropriate investigation of jaundice starts with a history of associated symptoms, and risk factors for liver disease.

H. The best part is that most infants with hyperbilirubinemia and associated jaundice recover without medical treatment.

6. Read the words in the box and finish the exercises after it.

> *Definition paragraph explains what a term or concept means. In a definition paragraph, you explain something to the reader: an unfamiliar term, concept, or a cultural event etc. You can do this by likening it to something your audience is familiar with, or by giving synonyms and explanations for it.*

1) Circle the term to be defined and underline the explanation.

Neonatal jaundice is yellowish discoloration of the skin, conjunctiva, and sclera due to elevated serum or plasma bilirubin in the newborn period. The term jaundice is from the French word "jaune", which means yellow. Neonatal jaundice occurs because the baby's blood contains an excess of bilirubin, a yellow pigment of red blood cells. Neonatal jaundice is typically a mild and transient event. However, it may at times be a sign of a problem with the baby's feeding, level of hydration or red blood cells lifespan. Other rare causes such as metabolism disorders, gland malfunction or liver disease can also present with jaundice.

2) Reorder the following sentences to make an effective paragraph.

A. However, it may at times be a sign of a problem with the baby's feeding, level of hydration or red blood cells lifespan.

B. Neonatal jaundice describes a condition in which an infant's skin appears yellow within the first few days of life.

C. In many cases this is a normal process and occurs in about 2/3 of all healthy newborns.

D. In some cases, a specialist in liver disease or blood disorders may be called in to help take care of the newborn.

E. The yellowish appearance is a sign of an increased blood pigment called Bilirubin, which then settles in the skin.

F. Other rare causes such as metabolism disorders, gland malfunction, or liver disease can also present with jaundice.

G. The choice of treatment is made according to the severity of the jaundice, the cause for the increase of bilirubin or the type of bilirubin.

H. Only the health care provider can determine if the infant's jaundice is normal and may order a blood test to help with diagnosis.

I. Treatment can be very simple from increasing the baby's water intake and modifying the feeding to very complex treatment.

Answer: __ __ __ __ __ __ __ __ __

7. Translate the Chinese paragraph below into English.

新生儿黄疸是小儿在产后过渡期出现的正常生理现象，表现为皮肤、虹膜及其他组织上出现黄橙色的色素沉淀。新生儿黄疸的出现通常是由于新生儿血液中含有过量的胆红素。新生儿，尤其是早产儿的胆红素结合分泌系统还未发育完全。而在某些条件下，胆红素有一定毒性，所以医生需在新生儿出生一周内密切监测其胆红素水平。

8. Read the text and fill in the sheet with proper information.

Reading Prompts	
Items	**Your Answers**
1) Identify the medical terms concerning **neonatal jaundice** and group them according to your understanding.	
2) Identify the **adjectives** used in "**Epidemiology**" and explain what conditions they describe.	
3) Identify the **prepositions** used in "**Prolonged jaundice**" and point out the logical relation each of them indicates.	
4) Identify the **verbs** used in "**Phototherapy**" and point out the changes of verb tenses.	
5) Identify the **typical sentence patterns**. (the whole article)	
6) Identify the **topic sentence** and the **supporting sentences** in paragraph 2 in "Management".	

Title: _____

A child is the most important person in a parent's life for whom they care most. Everybody wants to keep his or her children healthy, fit and free from illness. There are various aspects of the word "Health": it includes physical and mental domains as well as prevention from infections, allergies and injuries. Here are several tips for practitioners to follow and keep a watch on child's health and ways to improve it.

Ensure Breastfeeding

Breastfeeding is the first step to promote the health of a baby. Breastfeeding the baby has numerous benefits. Exclusive breastfeeding has shown to reduce morbidity and mortality from infectious illness during the first two years of life. Breast milk consists of numerous antibodies and enzymes which enhance the immune system of the child and protects against infections and allergies. Breastfeeding is also important for the neurological development of the child.

Maintaining Healthy Weight

Body mass index (BMI) is one of the most important tools to assess if a child's growth is normal or not. It shows the relationship between weight as well as height of the child and is a better tool than following only the weight of the child. The weight of a child depends upon diet, physical activity and sleep.

• Diet

Diet of a child influences his/her growth, and is one of the most important factors affecting health during childhood. A balanced diet supplies calories in the form of protein, carbohydrates and fats, as well as minerals and vitamins, which are all important for maintaining health of a child. Children who receive a proper diet remain healthier in the long term, free from various diseases and deficiencies.

Breast milk is the ideal food for a newborn provided by the mother. WHO advocates exclusive breastfeeding for the first six months of life and it should be continued until 2 years of age. Semi-solids and solids should be introduced to infants six months onwards. Try to add different varieties of food slowly till the age of one year, after which the child is usually able to eat all the home cooked foods. Homemade foods are preferable to commercially available formula foods as there are concerns of high sodium and sugar content in many commercially prepared foods which may cause harm to babies.

A balanced diet consists of carbohydrates, proteins, vitamins, and minerals and meets the daily caloric needs of the body.

The diet of a child must have a variety of foods from different sources of vitamins, minerals, proteins and fibers. Dairy and poultry products are rich sources of energy, calcium and protein, while foods such as cereals, vegetables and fruits provide energy as well as minerals, vitamins and fibers. It is very important to maintain adequate hydration, so offer plenty of water.

• Promoting regular physical activity

Young children and adolescents should engage in physical activity on a regular basis. Regular physical activity improves strength and endurance, keeps bones healthy, helps in maintaining weight and BMI, prevents hypertension, high cholesterol level and many chronic diseases like asthma and various cancers, improves immunity, promotes mental health, and even improves academic performance of children.

Children can engage in various kinds of physical activities, which improve their cardiovascular or aerobic fitness, strength and endurance, exercises which improve flexibility and provide better motor coordination.

• Promoting adequate sleep

Sleep plays a vital role for the health of a child. Adequate sleep is important for the physical as well as mental health of children. During sleep, new pathways are formed in the brain that helps in the maintenance of learning and memory. A good night's sleep is also important for proper attention and decision-making. Sleep deficiency in children can make them angry and impulsive, hyperactive and can affect their performance in school. Sleep is also necessary for physical health of children. During sleep, hormones are secreted which promote growth of body and repair of body tissues. Deep sleep also maintains balance of appetite controlling hormones. Sleep deficiency has been reported as a causal factor in the development of obesity in children and teens. Adequate sleep is also important for maintenance of immune function of the body.

Ensure Timely Immunization

Immunization is one of the most effective ways of protecting a child from serious diseases. By immunizing a child, the child is saved from developing that disease and at the same time the spread of that disease in community is also prevented.

Promoting Oral Health

Dental caries and tooth decay are common problems encountered in children which can affect a child's health and quality of life. Tooth decay can cause pain and discomfort, interfere with sleep and eating, and make them irritable.

Promoting Mental Health

The mental health of a child is equally important as the physical health of a child and it should be addressed carefully at each healthcare visit. Mental health can be affected due to various factors like any chronic illness in the child or any family member, disharmony among family members, maternal depression, genetic factors causing congenital developmental delay, or skill deficiency. Tips that can maintain or promote mental health of a child are:

□ *a warm and supportive relationship between parents and child*

□ *promoting self-esteem of the child*

□ *helping in development of coping skills*

□ *promoting peer relationships*

□ *communicating with child frequently—it helps the child to articulate feelings and problems faced by him*

□ *maintaining a family environment*

(Extracted from https://link.springer.com)

Exercises

1. **Read the article and write a possible title for it.**

2. **Answer the following questions according to the passage.**

   1) What is the topic of the article based on the first paragraph?

   2) How does breastfeeding benefit babies?

   3) What is a healthy diet for children?

   4) How can regular physical activities benefit children?

   5) What efforts can be made to provide a healthy environment for children in your opinion?

UNIT 10 Cardiology

Cardiovascular diseases names a group of disorders of heart and blood vessels, including hypertension (high blood pressure), coronary heart disease (heart attack), cerebrovascular disease (stroke), peripheral vascular disease and heart failure etc. Cardiovascular disease remains the leading cause of death globally.

Part I Intensive Reading

Coronary Artery Disease

Coronary artery diseases (CAD) are also known as atherosclerotic heart disease, atherosclerotic cardiovascular disease, coronary heart disease (CHD), or ischemic heart disease. It is the most common type of heart disease worldwide. Myocardial infarction is still the first common manifestation of it and, in about 50% of patients, angina pectoris is the first symptom of the pathology.

Epidemiology

The 20th century was the first century in which heart disease was the most common cause of death in the US, and it may be the last century during which it was the leading cause of death. Heart disease was uncommon in the early years of the 20th century. In 1900, it was the fourth most common cause of death, trailing infectious diseases such as pneumonia and tuberculosis. Three decades later, heart disease deaths had increased to become the commonest cause of death in the US. Heart disease deaths continued to increase until the mid-1960s. The large majority of cardiac deaths in the US are due to coronary heart disease secondary to coronary atherosclerosis. In 2009, coronary heart disease accounted for 64% of all cardiac deaths.

Many explanations for the increase in coronary heart disease deaths from 1900 to the 1960s have been offered. The marked increase in deaths attributed to heart disease, from 1900 until the late 1960s, was almost certainly due to an increase in the incidence of coronary atherosclerosis, with resultant coronary heart disease. Americans were living longer due to a decrease in deaths from infectious diseases. Changes in diet led to the consumption of processed foods, more saturated fats, added sugars and other high glycemic index carbohydrates. There was a spectacular increase in cigarette smoking: <5% of Americans were smokers in 1900, compared with 42% in 1965. Others point to a decrease in exercise and regular physical activity as most Americans gained access to automobiles.

Mechanisms/Pathophysiology

Atherosclerosis, the underlying cause of coronary heart disease (CHD), is a chronic inflammatory condition involving the subendothelial layer of coronary as well as other large and medium-sized arteries. This disease process is initiated early in life by multiple risk factors. Endothelial dysfunction and lipid infiltration are fundamental for the initiation and progression of the atherosclerotic process. After many asymptomatic decades, acute coronary syndromes are generally triggered by a coronary occlusion, caused by a thrombosis initiated by disruption of a vulnerable lipid-laden plaque with a thin and noncalcified fibrosis cap. Epidemiology studies over the past 50 years have consistently observed an inverse association between CHD and regular physical activity and/or cardiorespiratory fitness. Supporting evidence of causative relationships has been provided by exercise training studies demonstrating multiple, plausible, cardioprotective and biological mechanisms. These pleotropic effects may be classified as: (1) direct antiatherosclerotic effects and indirect effects via reduction of other risk factors; (2) anti-ischemic effects by decreasing myocardial oxygen demands and increasing its vascular supply and by decreasing the severity of ischemic injuries by direct conditioning effects on cardiomyocytes; (3) antiarrhythmic effects by improving electrical stability of the heart; and (4) antithrombotic (and prothrombolytic) effects, reducing risk of a coronary thrombotic occlusion. It is concluded based on an impressive body of evidence that regular aerobic exercise attenuates the risk of CHD at all stages of the atherothrombotic process.

Diagnosis

- Clinical syndromes

Coronary atherosclerosis begins in adolescence and its initial alterations date back to childhood. However, its clinical manifestations only show up during adulthood, more frequently from the fourth decade of life on. It may then be concluded that the disease presents a long period of silent evolution before the manifestation of clinical CI, which can take various forms, as listed below.

Stable angina. Repeated anginal attacks, which can develop over months or years, are referred to as stable angina. An increase in myocardial oxygen consumption, usually due to physical exertion or emotions, triggers ischemia. It is relieved by rest or the use of vasodilators.

Heart failure. Heart failure associated with CAD is mainly due to two conditions—ischemic cardiomyopathy and aneurysm.

Silent ischemia (SI). About 3% of the normal population and 30% of asymptomatic patients experience silent ischemia following an infarction of the myocardium.

Acute coronary ischemia. Unstable angina, non Q-wave infarction, and infarction with Q-wave are characteristics of acute coronary ischemia.

Sudden death (SD). Approximately 1/3 of CAD patients die of SD, which can be due to primary malignant arrhythmias, such as ventricular tachycardia degenerating into ventricular fibrillation or ventricular fibrillation associated with acute ischemia.

Coronary disease in women. CAD in women occurs about 10 years later than it does in men. This is attributed to the protective effects of female hormones during the women's reproductive years.

- Diagnosis

A clinical history may provide important information for the diagnosis of CAD. Anginal pain, fatigue, dyspnea and palpitations are the most common complaints. Typical angina is the most easily diagnosed. Identification of triggering and relief factors, its duration and characteristic location and irradiation are indispensable for the diagnosis of typical angina. However, physical examination usually adds little to the diagnosis. Except in instances of heart failure, the physical examination is noticed only for being normal, which ironically contrasts with the potentially lethal situation.

Non-invasive examinations. Technical aspects will not be discussed here, but only several peculiarities of major interest to the cardiologist in general.

Electrocardiogram at rest. Most patients with heart failure are within normal standards. However, the presence of inactive areas suggesting a previous infarction, inverted T-waves, downslope of the ST segment and left ventricular hypertrophy are associated with a higher cardiovascular mortality rate in the long-range. The presence of extrasystoles, mainly those of ventricular origin, may suggest coronary disease. Both atrial-ventricular and fascicular condition disorders may occur, but these do not contribute to the detection of coronary disease because they are unspecific.

ECG stress test (ST). ST is very useful in tracking and stratifying coronary atherosclerotic disease and has an excellent level of reliability.

Radioisotopes. The versatility of radioisotopes allows them to be used to detect ischemia, fibrosis and to evaluate the LV mechanical function.

Resting and stress echocardiogram. The resting echocardiogram has considerable application in the diagnostic and non-invasive prognostic determination of the coronary atherosclerotic disease.

Echocardiogram with the use of micro-bubbles. The technical hindrance to the use of micro-bubbles is the low commercial availability.

Coronary angiography. The definitive exam for the diagnosis of coronary obstructive atherosclerosis is coronary angiography.

Magnetic resonance imaging. Magnetic resonance imaging (MRI) has been used in two instances to evaluate patients with coronary atherosclerotic disease—cellular metabolic study and cardiac form and function.

Management

The great options for CAD treatment include clinical/medicinal treatment, angioplasty and surgical revascularization. The clinical treatment is obviously always used, as neither percutaneous transluminal coronary angioplasty nor surgical revascularization interferes in the metabolic process of the basic disease.

- Clinical treatment

Nitrates. Nitrates are prodrugs that need to be converted into nitric oxide in the endothelial and smooth muscle cells in order to achieve their vasodilating effects.

Beta-blockers. Beta-blockers are efficient drugs for the treatment of angina, especially useful in effort angina.

Calcium channel antagonists. Ca++ ions are essential for contraction of the cardiac muscle and the vascular smooth muscle. Ca++ blockers represent a heterogeneous group of substances that block the movement of the Ca++ ions through the slow channels of the cellular membranes in cardiac and smooth muscle cells.

Angiotensin-converting enzyme inhibitors. Angiotensin-converting enzyme inhibitors prevent the conversion of angiotensin I to angiotensin II in circulation. Their hemodynamic actions are due to arterial vasodilation, which increase cardiac output; they also act on the lung and venous beds, reducing the pre-load.

Aspirin. Platelets play an important role in triggering acute coronary episodes and in the growth of atherosclerotic lesions.

Treatment of the underlying disease. The treatment of the underlying disease of atherosclerosis requires extensive life style changes by people who have known and modifiable risk factors. It is well known that arterial hypertension, a sedentary life, emotional stress, active and passive smoking, dyslipidemia, and obesity must be controlled. Moderate and continuous physical exercise should be encouraged.

Antioxidants and vitamins. Oxidative stress plays an important role in the pathophysiology of atherosclerosis.

Estrogens. Estrogens show obvious evidence of lowering the prevalence and incidence of coronary atherosclerosis in women in their reproductive years.

Genetic predisposition and CAD treatment. Undoubtedly, a family history of CAD, showing genetic predisposition to the disease, is a weighty risk factor. Genetic predisposition is present in approximately 20% of CAD cases.

Coronary angioplasty. Coronary angioplasty has been shown to have a similar effect as surgery and clinical treatment on the incidence of death or infarction. Compared with surgery, it is associated with a higher need of new procedures, especially in the first year post-intervention. However, after this initial phase the evolution is very good. An important advance has been the use of stents, intracoronary expansible prostheses, which have increased the frequency of the primary success and reduced the incidence of restenosis following hospital discharge.

Myocardial revascularization surgery. Revascularization is widely indicated, as an elective procedure, for thousands of patients due to its confirmed reduction of symptoms and increase in survival rates in certain subgroups.

Suggestions for practical approaches. Some general guidelines for the treatment of those at risk for CAD can be outlined: (1) middle-aged men and women should be evaluated for CAD risk, since the disease has a silent evolutionary period; (2) sons and daughters of CAD patients should be checked even earlier, preferably during adolescence, as the disease starts very early and has a strong family trend; (3) when patients are suspected of having CAD because of important risk factors or history suggestive of angina, non-invasive tests should be performed, such as ECG stress test, radioisotopes, or stress echocardiogram; (4) coronary angiography should be performed when suspicion of CAD exists based on clinical history or non-invasive tests; (5) women should be checked as carefully as men, naturally respecting certain peculiarities related to sex; (6) the choice of form of treatment should take into account the current knowledge about the CAD natural history, prognostic determinants, efficiency of the treatments available and individual conditions of the patients, such as age, associated diseases and occupation; (7) in the case of invasive treatments, the experience and competence of the local services are fundamentally important; (8) notwithstanding the form of treatment, one must remember that CAD is basically a progressive metabolic disease, whose control must be sought in the long-term. Recent information indicates that its natural course can be modified for the better by controlling risk factors.

Quality of Life

The QoL of patients with heart failure is poor despite advances in therapy. Of patients who survive the acute onset of heart failure, only 35% of men and 50% of women are alive after 5 years. Mortality rates are higher in older patients, men, and patients with a reduced left ventricular ejection fraction or underlying coronary heart disease.

Prevention

The prevention studies have shown that it is possible to alter the material course of atherosclerosis, decreasing its progression and even inducing plaque regression. Nevertheless, great challenges still persist: the identification of the real causes of atherosclerosis, early detection of lesions prone to destabilization, correct quantification of the degree of stenosis, the most efficient and safest treatment of the acute cases, and mainly the control of the underlying disease, atherosclerosis.

(Extracted from https://www.scielo.br)

Vocabulary

atherosclerotic	[ˌæθərəʊsklə'rɒtɪk]	*adj.*	动脉粥样硬化的
ischemic	[ɪs'kimɪk]	*adj.*	局部缺血的
myocardial	[ˌmaɪə'kaːdiəl]	*adj.*	心肌的
infarction	[ɪn'faːkʃn]	*n.*	梗塞形成；梗死形成
angina pectoris			心绞痛
glycemic	[glɪ'semɪk]	*adj.*	血糖的
thrombosis	[θrɒm'bəʊsɪs]	*n.*	血栓症
subendothelial	[sʌbendɒ'θiːlɪəl]	*adj.*	内皮下的

endothelial	[ˌendəʊ'θiːlɪəl]	*adj.* 内皮的
cardiorespiratory	[ˌkɑːdɪəʊrɪs'paɪərətərɪ]	*adj.* 心肺的
aneurysm	['ænjərɪzəm]	*n.* 动脉瘤
vasodilator	[ˌveɪzəʊdaɪ'leɪtə]	*n.* 血管扩张神经
palpitation	[ˌpælpɪ'teɪʃən]	*n.* 心悸
ventricular	[ven'trɪkjələ(r)]	*adj.* 心室的；膨胀的
hypertrophy	[haɪ'pɜːtrəfɪ]	*n.* 肥大；过度生长
extrasystole	[ˌekstrə'sɪstəliː]	*n.* 期前收缩；额外收缩
fascicular	[fə'sɪkjʊlə(r)]	*adj.* 成束的
versatility	[ˌvɜːsə'tɪlətɪ]	*n.* 多功能性
radioisotope	[ˌreɪdɪəʊ'aɪsətəʊp]	*n.* 放射性同位元素
angioplasty	['ændʒɪəʊplæstɪ]	*n.* 血管成形术
transluminal	[træns'lʊːmɪnəl]	*adj.* 穿过（血管）腔壁的
nitrate	['naɪtreɪt]	*n.* 硝酸盐
prodrug	['prəʊˌdrʌg]	*n.* 前药
hemodynamic	[ˌhemədaɪ'næmɪk]	*adj.* 血液动力学的
vasodilation	[ˌveɪzəʊdaɪ'leɪʃn]	*n.* 血管舒张
dyslipidemia	[dɪslɪpɪ'demɪə]	*n.* 血脂障碍

Exercises

1. Read the text and explain the following medical phrases.

1）Alternative names of CAD

2）Pathophysiology of CHD

3）Clinical syndromes of coronary atherosclerosis

4）Diagnosis of CAD

5）Management of CAD

2. Answer the following questions according to the text.

1）Why did CHD deaths increase from 1900 to the 1960s?

2）How does CHD relate to regular physical activity?

3）What is the syndrome of coronary disease in women? And why?

4）How does a doctor treatthe underlying disease of atherosclerosis?

3. Fill in the blanks with the proper forms of the given words.

block	buildup	artery	arrhythmia	narrow
chest	oxygen	harden	plaque	noticeable

Coronary heart disease, the most common type of heart disease, is when 1)_____ builds up in the arteries leading to the heart. CHD is also called coronary 2)_____ disease (CAD). When arteries narrow, the heart cannot get enough blood and 3)_____. A 4)_____ artery can cause a heart attack. Over time, CHD can weaken the heart muscle and cause heart failure or 5)_____. CHD is the leading cause of death in the United States for men and women. CHD is caused by the 6)_____ of plaque in the arteries to one's heart. This may also be called 7)_____. Fatty material and other substances can form a plaque buildup on the walls of the coronary arteries which bring blood and oxygen to heart. This buildup causes the arteries to get 8)_____. As a result, blood flow to the heart can slow down or stop. In some cases, symptoms may be very 9)_____. But, you can have the disease and not have any symptoms. This is more often true in the early stages of heart disease. 10)_____ pain or discomfort (angina) is the most common symptom. You feel this pain when the heart is not getting enough blood or oxygen. The pain may feel different from person to person.

4. **Study the bold-faced words in each of the following sentences and imitate the particular way of writing.**

Mentor Sentence:

☆ In morbidly obese patients, bariatric surgery **can be an effective means of** weight loss.

Imitation Sentence:

☆ Parenteral vaccination **can be an effective means of** inducing protective mucosal responses.

1) **The large majority of** cardiac deaths **in** the US **are due to** coronary heart disease **secondary to** coronary atherosclerosis.

Answer: **The large majority of** _____ **in** _____ **are due to** _____
_____ **secondary to** _____

2) The large majority of cardiac deaths in the US are **due to** coronary heart disease secondary to coronary atherosclerosis. In 2009 coronary heart disease **accounted for** 64% of all cardiac deaths.

Answer: _____ **due to** _____

_____

accounted for _____

3) There was a spectacular increase in cigarette smoking: <5% of Americans were smokers in 1900, **compared with** 42% in 1965.

Answer: _____ ,

compared with _____

4) **It is well known that** arterial hypertension, a sedentary life, emotional stress, active and passive smoking, dyslipidemia, and obesity **must be controlled.**

Answer: **It is well known that** _____

_____ **must be controlled.**

5. Match the following statements with the corresponding sections in the text.

Epidemiology: _____   Management: _____

Mechanisms/Pathophysiology: _____   Quality of Life: _____

Diagnosis: _____   Prevention: _____

A. The large majority of cardiac deaths in the US are due to coronary heart disease secondary to coronary atherosclerosis.

B. In 2009 coronary heart disease accounted for 64% of all cardiac deaths.

C. The marked increase in deaths attributed to heart disease, from 1900 until the late 1960s, was almost certainly due to an increase in the incidence of coronary atherosclerosis, with resultant coronary heart disease.

D. Coronary atherosclerosis begins in adolescence and its initial alterations date back to childhood.

E. However, its clinical manifestations only show up during adulthood, more frequently from the fourth decade of life on.

F. Anginal pain, fatigue, dyspnea, and palpitations are the most common complaints.

G. Typical angina is the most easily diagnosed.

H. Identification of triggering and relief factors, its duration and characteristic location and irradiation are indispensable for the diagnosis of typical angina.

I. Atherosclerosis is a chronic inflammatory condition involving the subendothelial layer of coronary as well as other large- and medium-sized arteries.

J. This disease process is initiated early in life by multiple risk factors.

K. Endothelial dysfunction and lipid infiltration are fundamental for the initiation and progression of the atherosclerotic process.

L. The health-related quality of life significantly changed from one to three years after the treatment in the patients with CAD.

M. While the physical health deteriorated during the two-year follow-up, mental health improved at the same time.

N. The great options for CAD treatment include clinical or medicinal treatment, angioplasty and surgical revascularization.

O. The prevention studies have shown that it is possible to alter the material course of atherosclerosis, decreasing its progression and even inducing plaque regression.

6. Read the introduction in the box and finish the exercises after it.

> ***Enumeration*** *is a writing device used for listing details. Writers use enumeration to elucidate a topic, to make it understandable for the readers. In this type of paragraph development, topic sentences are often used to introduce a list of items. Such paragraphs, based on a pattern of enumeration, have topic sentences that typically include quantifiers, such as **numerous**, **several**, **many**, **much** and **a number of**. For example, there are **a number of** good reasons for physical exercises.*

1) Underline the list of items.

The doctor may recommend one or more of the following tests to assist the diagnosis of coronary artery disease: electrocardiography, stress test, echocardiography, blood tests, coronary angiography and cardiac catheterization. Electrocardiography can show signs of heart damage due to CAD and signs of a previous or current heart attack. Stress test can show possible signs and symptoms of CAD, such as abnormal changes in your heart rate or blood pressure. Echocardiography also can show areas of poor blood flow to the heart, areas of heart muscle that aren't contracting normally, and previous injury to the heart muscle caused by poor blood flow. Blood tests check the levels of certain fats, cholesterol, sugar, and proteins in your blood. Coronary angiography and cardiac catheterization use dye and special X-rays to show the insides of your coronary arteries.

2) Reorder the following sentences to make an effective paragraph.

A. Stable Angina: stable angina is the most common type of angina which occurs when the heart is working harder than usual and has a regular pattern.

B. This is because they have different symptoms and require different treatments.

C. The major types of angina are stable, unstable, variant, and microvascular.

D. Knowing how the types differ is important.

E. Microvascular Angina: microvascular angina can be more severe and last longer than other types of angina.

F. Unstable Angina: unstable angina does not follow a pattern which may occur more often, be more severe than stable angina or can occur with or without physical exertion.

G. Variant Angina: variant angina is rare and usually occurs at rest; the pain can be severe.

Answer:__ __ __ __ __ __ __

7. Translate the Chinese paragraph below into English.

冠状动脉粥样硬化性心脏病是冠状动脉血管发生动脉粥样硬化病变而引起血管腔狭窄或阻塞,造成心肌缺血、缺氧或坏死而导致的心脏病,常常被称为"冠心病"。但是冠心病的范围可能更广泛,还包括炎症、栓塞等导致管腔狭窄或闭塞。

8. Read the text and fill in the sheet with proper information.

Reading Prompts	
Items	**Your Answers**
1) *Identify those medical terms concerning* **CAD** *and group them according to your understanding.*	
2) *Identify the* **adjectives** *used in* **"Epidemiology"** *and explain what conditions they describe.*	
3) *Identify the* **conjunctions** *used in the text and point out the logical relation each of them indicates.*	
4) *Identify the* **verbs** *used in* **"Management"** *and point out the changes of verb tenses.*	
5) *Identify the* **typical sentence patterns.** (*the whole article*)	
6) *Identify the* **topic sentence** *and the* **supporting sentences in paragraph 2 in "Epidemiology".**	

Title: _____

Alfred Nobel discovered dynamite and became one of the richest men in the world by manufacturing armaments. When a younger brother died in France in 1888, French newspapers mistakenly thought it was Alfred. Their headlines read "The Merchant of Death is Dead". The papers declared that Alfred's powerful explosives killed more people more efficiently than ever before. The incident had a profound effects on him. He began thinking how he could leave a positive legacy. After his death in 1896, his will created a foundation from his enormous estate that would bestow prizes to individuals who had achieved significant benefits for humankind. The fields of Medicine, Physics, Chemistry, Literature, and Peace were singled out. The Nobel Prize has become identified as the most coveted in the world.

In 1956, the Prize in Medicine was awarded to the developers of cardiac catheterization, Drs André Cournand and Dickinson Richards from America and Dr Werner Forssmann from Germany. Who were these men, and what was their accomplishment? André Cournand was born in Paris in 1895. He graduated from medical school in 1925 and then spent six years working in pulmonary disease clinics. In 1931, he migrated to New York, having received an appointment as a resident in the Columbia's Chest Service at Bellevue Hospital. He made friends with Dickinson Richards there.

Dickinson Richards was born in New Jersey in 1895. He graduated from Columbia's medical school in 1923. After several years of training on the Chest Service at Bellevue he met André Cournand. They bonded immediately as close friends and worked productively as a team. In 1940, they read an intriguing article in an obscure German medical journal written 11 years previously by Werner Forssmann. The subject was catheterization of the human heart. They realized the enormous potential of cardiac catheterization.

In 1929, Werner Forssmann was a general practitioner in a small town near Berlin. He was interested in the problems of heart diseases and speculated on the effectiveness of administering digitalis directly into the heart. Operating on a dog, he inserted a urological catheter through a leg vein into the right atrium. The dog survived. He became obsessed with the idea of doing the same thing on a human, but his colleagues at his hospital thought his idea was insane. They forbade him to do the experiment on a person. He determined to perform heart catheterization on himself and convinced the operating room nurse at the hospital to cooperate with him. She agreed, but with the stipulation that he would catheterize himself, not her. One Sunday, he went through the motions of starting the procedure on her. Instead, he isolated his own left antecubital vein and threaded the catheter into his upper chest. He then told the nurse what he had done and asked her to call an X-ray technician to the X-ray room. They walked down two flights of stairs to the X-ray department, and, once there, he advanced the catheter a total of 65 cm from the elbow. An X-ray showed the catheter well into his heart. There were no ill effects, and the catheter was removed. Forssmann did not follow up on his experiment. In 1932, he joined the Nazi party and remained a member until 1945.

Cournand and Richards planned to follow-up on Forssmann's idea but the entry into World War II made them postpone their plans. They worked on the problem of traumatic shock with relevance to the war effort. In 1945, they confirmed Forssmann's experiment and opened a cardiac catheterization laboratory at Bellevue Hospital. It was an immediate success. Details of heart and lung dysfunction were disclosed and many publications were written. In 1948, Dr John R. West became a valuable member of the team. A brilliant researcher, he designed and constructed most of the recording equipment in the laboratory. In 1951, a second laboratory was opened at Presbyterian Hospital, directed by Dr West. This time, I was interviewed by Dr West and gained the assignment to work mornings in his laboratory.

My time in the laboratory was a marvelous learning experience with Dr West, who was charismatic and passionate about his work. I learned to use the catheters, perform arterial punctures, use a fluoroscope, and analyze pulmonary function data. Early in 1954, we were devastated to learn that Dr John West was diagnosed with leukemia. In June, at age 37, he died of a cerebral hemorrhage. Dr Richards wrote a touching obituary, stressing a great scientific potential that would never be fully realized.

The great contribution to humanity made by the "cath lab" was recognized in 1956 when the Nobel Prize in medicine was awarded to Drs Cournand, Richards and Forssmann. Through a remarkable chain of events, my wife and I were able to attend the awards ceremony in Stockholm and to cheer loudly for them. It was an unforgettable evening. White tie, tails, ribbons for the men, evening gowns and jewels for the women. The walls of the opera house were covered with blue and yellow flowers, colors of the Swedish flag. The king of Sweden spoke to each recipient in French and English. After each presentation, the full orchestra played a short piece. It was a spectacular production, a once-in-a-lifetime occasion.

(Extracted from *Journal of Vascular Surgery*)

Exercises

1. **Read the article and write a possible title for it.**

2. **Answer the following questions according to the passage.**

   1) What did the headline "The Merchant of Death is Dead" mean?

   2) Who won the Prize in Medicine in 1956? And why?

   3) What did Richards and Cournand realize after reading the intriguing article?

   4) What was Werner Forssmann's insane behavior in 1929?

   5) What has the author learned from Dr West?

UNIT 11 Gastroenterology

Gastroenterology studies physiology and pathology of esophagus, stomach, small intestine, colon and rectum, pancreas, gallbladder, bile ducts and liver. Common gastrointestinal disorders include celiac disease, constipation, diarrhea and irritable bowel syndrome.

Part I Intensive Reading

Irritable Bowel Syndrome

The irritable bowel syndrome (IBS) is a functional gastrointestinal disorder whose hallmark is abdominal pain or discomfort associated with a change in the consistency or frequency of stools. It is one of over 20 functional gastrointestinal (GI) tract disorders characterized by chronic or recurrent GI tract symptoms that are not explained by structural abnormalities, infection, or metabolic changes.

Epidemiology

Epidemiological data are based on diagnostic criteria. Although IBS has historically been diagnosed by exclusion, expert working teams originally developed "positive" symptom criteria, known as the Rome criteria. The Rome criteria have led to greater uniformity in epidemiological studies of IBS and have facilitated comparisons among population subgroups. Estimates of the prevalence of IBS among adults are based on population surveys. Most surveys have been conducted in developed countries and reflect the prevalence of IBS in those cultures. The prevalence of GI symptoms and functional diagnoses is similar in many countries. In the western world, 8%-23% of adults have IBS or other functional GI symptoms, and approximately 60%-70% of these are women. IBS is also common in Asia and Africa. In India and Sri Lanka, the gender ratio is reversed with a predominance of male patients, possibly reflecting sociological differences in gender patterns of symptom reporting and health care utilization. Preliminary data from an epidemiological study in Israel and the Palestinian Authorities indicate a similar trend among Palestinian adults. As recently hypothesized, there may be socialized gender roles or differential male and female traits that contribute to the difference in gender prevalence of IBS in various cultures.

The syndrome of recurrent abdominal pain begins in childhood and tracks into adulthood as IBS. Symptoms of IBS wax and wane throughout life, but the majority of patients seen by physicians are in the 20- to 50-year age range. Absenteeism rates from work or school are significantly higher among patients with IBS than among normal individuals. The cost of health services for patients with IBS is significantly higher than for controls in the United States.

Mechanisms/Pathophysiology

- Pathophysiology

The pathophysiology of IBS is incompletely understood, although research over the past several years has shed light on a variety of putative pathophysiological mechanisms that allow us to synthesize a more integrated understanding of IBS as a brain-gut disorder. A review of IBS research over the past half century shows a changing focus from psychological and stress-related research to an emphasis on motility disturbances to autonomic system imbalance and visceral hypersensitivity. In recent years, research has centered on the dysregulation of brain-gut interactions as the pathophysiological basis for IBS. The experience of abdominal pain and/or altered motility and bowel habits can derive from dysregulation of activity in one or more of the stations in the bidirectional communication pathways between the GI system (the enteric nervous system) and the spinal cord and brain.

The brain-gut dysregulation. The brain-gut dysregulation in IBS may be triggered by several kinds of events. Among these are psychological experiences, such as life stress, psychological comorbidity, or sexual and physical abuse, and inflammatory structural events, such as acute gastroenteritis or other causes of transient or chronic inflamed intestinal mucosa. The common factor in these occurrences is an insult that leads to a hypothesized "chronic memory state" with reduced thresholds for pain and other symptom experiences, all mediated through brain-gut interactions with varying contributions from brain and gut.

Mucosal inflammation. Mucosal inflammation may play a role in the development of IBS in some cases. Inflammation can lead to increased cytokine activity, motility, or release of 5HT (5-hydroxytryptamine), all of which can upregulate pain sensation. This may be mediated through activation of silent nociceptors at the mucosal/myenteric plexus level, through upregulation or "wind-up" of afferent neurotransmission at the level of the dorsal horn or at the level of the brain.

Psychosocial factors. Even though psychosocial factors do not define functional bowel disorders and are not required for their diagnosis, they do modulate patients' behaviors and illness experience and have a major effects on clinical outcomes, such as quality of life, physician visits, and use of medication. Indeed, it has been shown that severe IBS can be differentiated from moderate IBS more by behavioral/psychosocial features than by mechanisms such as visceral hypersensitivity.

- Disease chronicity and exacerbations

As a chronic, functional disorder, IBS may be associated with changes in mood, particularly depression and anxiety. However, psychological distress as evidenced in subjective psychological and personality testing may not be indicative of a depression disorder or serious psychiatric pathology. Anxiety and depression, which upregulate symptoms among many patients with IBS, can be associated with a "vicious cycle": the effects of living with chronic discomforting and disabling symptoms, along with the frustration of not understanding the nature of the disorder and of being misunderstood by physicians and/or members of close family and social circles, can in turn lead to worsening of symptoms.

- Risk factors

Genetics. Many patients with IBS report having relatives who share their diagnosis or who report similar symptoms, and indeed studies have observed familial aggregation of IBS, suggesting an underlying genetic component. Nonetheless, findings are confounded by the fact that, within families, individuals will often have shared childhood experiences or environmental exposures in common, which might equally explain clustering of IBS symptomology.

Dietary factors. Patients frequently report dietary triggers for their IBS symptoms and a western diet high in sugar and fat has been associated with IBS. Patients with IBS might have lactose malabsorption, although the relevance of this suggestion is questionable given the poor response of symptoms to a lactose-free diet and similar prevalence of lactose malabsorption in people with no IBS symptoms.

The gut microbiome. Interest has been growing into the role that the gut microbiome, with a particular focus on bacteria, might play in health and gastrointestinal disease. Researches show that the fecal microbiota of people with IBS differs significantly from that of healthy individuals and might influence colonic transit, which further alter bowel habits.

Post-infection IBS. Infective gastroenteritis is frequently identified as a risk factor for developing IBS. Such patients generally experience looser and more frequent stools rather than constipations. Early studies determined that a quarter of individuals with infective gastroenteritis reported persistence of altered bowel habits 6 months after their infective episode, with 1 in 14 people developing IBS.

Psychological comorbidity. Psychological comorbidity, including stress, anxiety, or depression, is frequently associated with IBS and might exacerbate symptoms. It is important to consider that psychological symptoms might have developed as a consequence of the severity and effects of IBS on an individual, or might instead have been present prior to the onset of gastrointestinal symptoms.

Diagnosis

Abdominal pain or discomfort, associated with a change in the consistency or frequency of stools and relieved by defecation, is the hallmark of IBS. The abdominal pain/discomfort is often poorly localized and may be migratory and variable in nature. However, it often occurs after a meal, during psychological stress, or at the time of menses. Altered bowel habit (i. e. diarrhea or constipation) is also common in patients with IBS. Associated symptoms can include bloating or a feeling of distention, mucus in the stool, urgency, a feeling of incomplete evacuation, or other GI symptoms such as heartburn, nausea, dyspepsia or early satiety.

The initial evaluation involves a detailed patient history. According to the understanding of IBS as a biopsychosocial disorder, patient evaluation should include careful description of physical symptoms related to the patient's psychosocial wellbeing. The psychosocial aspects of the illness are an essential part of the patient's evaluation and need to be understood as predisposing, precipitating, and perpetuating factors. The psychosocial history should be elicited within the framework of the physical symptom history and the patient should be encouraged to tell the story in his or her own way. This will allow better understanding of the symptoms in the context of the psychosocial events surrounding the illness.

Because symptoms alone are not fully specific for the diagnosis, it is necessary to exclude other medical disorders with similar clinical presentation. Certain symptoms/warning features should be regarded as alert signs or "red flag", since their presence can suggest a diagnosis other than IBS and require further evaluation. These include symptoms that awaken the patient from sleep, first presentation at an older age, GI bleeding, weight loss and fever. The initial evaluation should also include the following limited diagnostic screening tests: a complete blood count; a test of sedimentation rate; chemistries; tests of the stool for ova, parasites, and blood; and sigmoidoscopy. Colonoscopy or barium enema with sigmoidoscopy are recommended if the patient is older than 40 – 50 years. Other studies may be performed according to the patient's dominant symptom. For example, a lactose H2 breath test, thyroid-stimulating hormone, or celiac sprue serology may be appropriate for patients with diarrhea-predominant symptoms, or a plain abdominal radiograph during an acute episode may be useful for a patient with pain/gas/bloating. Additional studies depend on the patient's history, age of onset of symptoms, family history of colon cancer, change in symptoms over time (e. g. getting worse or better), previous diagnostic evaluations and psychosocial status.

Finally, if the initial screening evaluation is normal, the physician should withhold further diagnostic studies and begin treatment with a follow-up within 4 – 6 weeks. This allows the physician to reevaluate the patient's clinical status at two or three points in time before deciding on further diagnostic tests. In most cases, if the patient is better or not worse, studies can be withheld.

Management

The treatment approach depends on identifying and integrating several factors: the intensity, frequency, and constancy of the symptoms, the nature of the physiological disturbances (i. e. diarrhea or constipation), the degree of psychosocial difficulties and the frequency of health care utilization.

Many patients with IBS do not require prescription medications. They usually benefit from dietary changes, recommendations for lifestyle changes, and encouragement of health-promoting behaviors. Identifying offending dietary substances (e. g. lactose, caffeine, fatty foods, alcohol, gas-producing foods and sorbitol) and making dietary modifications can help some patients. Physicians should keep in mind that patients may attribute their symptoms to specific components of their diet and begin a process of dietary elimination that can lead to severely unbalanced nutrition or an obsessive preoccupation with diet. Recommendations for dietary changes should usually also involve lifestyle changes and encouragement of health-promoting behaviors. Short-term medication can be prescribed during exacerbations.

Quality of Life

While irritable bowel syndrome（IBS）is not life-threatening for most，it has enormous influence on quality of life and mental health. When patients come into contact with inducing factors in their daily life，especially under the influence of lifestyle and mental pressure，there is a greater chance of recurrence. Patients should pay attention to the inducing factors and record them. By avoiding these factors，they can effectively reduce the number of recurrence.

Prevention

Dietary changes，medications，and psychotherapy can help prevent IBS. Prevention measures include：
- *avoiding triggering foods*
- *increasing your fiber intake，which can relieve constipation*
- *exercising more*
- *getting enough sleep*
- *drinking enough fluids*
- *avoiding stressful situations*

If these simple steps aren't enough to control your symptoms，dietary changes may be worth considering.

（Extracted from https：//www. annualreviews. org）

Vocabulary

putative	['pjuːtətɪv]	adj. 推定的；认定的；公认的
visceral	['vɪsərəl]	adj. 内脏的
dysregulation	[dɪsregjʊ'leɪʃn]	n. 调节障碍；调节异常
comorbidity	[ˌkəʊmɒr'bɪdəti]	n. 疾病；伴随疾病
nociceptor	[ˌnəʊsɪ'septə(r)]	n. 伤害感受器；疼痛感受器
myenteric	[ˌmaɪen'terɪk]	adj. 肠肌层的
plexus	['pleksəs]	n. 神经丛
afferent	['æfərənt]	adj. 传入的；输入的
lactose	['læktəʊz]	n. 乳糖
malabsorption	[ˌmæləb'sɒrpʃn]	n. 吸收不良；吸收障碍
microbiota	[ˌmaɪkrəʊbaɪ'əʊtə]	n. 小型生物群
migratory	['maɪgrətrɪ]	adj. 迁移的
distention	[dɪs'tenʃn]	n. 膨胀；扩张

sedimentation	[sedɪmenˈteɪʃn]	n. 沉淀
sigmoidoscopy	[ˌsɪgmɔɪˈdɒskəpɪ]	n. 乙状结肠镜检查
celiac	[ˈsiːlɪæk]	adj. 腹的；腹腔的
sprue	[spruː]	n. 口炎性腹泻

Exercises

1. Read the text and explain the following medical phrases.

1) Hallmark of IBS

2) Pathophysiological basis for IBS

3) Risk factors for IBS

4) Guidelines to manage stable IBS

5) Prevention measures of IBS

2. Answer the following questions according to the text.

1) What can trigger brain-gut dysregulation in IBS?

2) How does mucosal inflammation work in developing IBS?

3) How does a doctor diagnose IBS?

4) What are the alert signs of IBS?

3. Fill in the blanks with the proper forms of the given words.

| undiagnose | gastrointestinal | perception | adherence | adjust |
| quantify | abdominal | diagnostic | assess | severity |

IBS is one of the gastrointestinal disorders. The disease is not life-threatening, but it is embarrassing to talk about and it often goes 1)_____. The causes of IBS are not clear, nor is there a cure for it. The general symptoms of IBS include 2)_____ pain, bloating, diarrhea and constipation. The challenge to assigning a degree of 3)_____ to an individual patient with IBS is generally compounded by a lack of a valid evidence for the disorder. Hence, severity is typically determined based on an 4)_____ of the patients' self-reported symptoms and behaviors. As a consequence, IBS and functional 5)_____ diseases, in general, are best understood from the patient's personal experience of ill health. Some patients with mild symptoms can control their symptoms by managing diet or lifestyle and stress. Others will need medication and counselling. Patients' 6)_____ to medications, 7)_____ of their lifestyles and pursuit of health care are based on their own 8)_____ of severity of the disease. Clinicians may not always take this into consideration. They

should weigh the patient's symptom reports and behaviors to make proper 9)____
____ and treatment decisions. Hence, doctors should 10) _____ and
understand the severity of the disease from the patient's perspective.

4. **Study the bold-faced words in each of the following sentences and imitate the particular way of writing.**

Mentor Sentence:

☆ In morbidly obese patients, bariatric surgery **can be an effective means of** weight loss.

Imitation Sentence:

☆ Parenteral vaccination **can be an effective means of** inducing protective mucosal responses.

1) The syndrome of recurrent abdominal pain **begins in** childhood and **tracks into** adulthood as IBS.

Answer: _____ **begins/begin in** _____ **and tracks/ track into** _____

2) The pathophysiology of IBS is incompletely understood, although research over the past several years has **shed light on** a variety of putative pathophysiological mechanisms that allow us to synthesize a more integrated understanding of IBS as a brain-gut disorder.

Answer: _____ **has/have shed light on** _____

_____

3) **The common factor in these occurrences is an insult that** leads to a hypothesized "chronic memory state" with reduced thresholds for pain and other symptom experiences, all mediated through brain-gut interactions, with varying contributions from brain and gut.

Answer: **The common factor in these occurrences is an insult that** _____

_____

4) **Indeed, it has been shown that** severe IBS **can be differentiated from** moderate IBS more by behavioral/psychosocial features than **by** mechanisms such as visceral hypersensitivity.

Answer: **Indeed, it has been shown that** _____ **can be differentiated from** _____ **by** _____

_____

5. **Match the following statements with the corresponding sections in the text.**

Epidemiology: _____ Management: _____

Mechanisms/Pathophysiology: _____   Quality of Life:_____

Diagnosis:_____   Prevention:_____

A. The experience of symptoms derives from dysregulation of the bidirectional communication system between the gastrointestinal tract and the brain, mediated by neuroendocrine and immunological factors and modulated by psychosocial factors.

B. In the western world, 8% to 23% of adults have IBS and its socioeconomic cost is substantial.

C. The diagnosis of IBS is based on recognizing clinical symptoms consistent with it and on modest efforts to exclude other/organic diseases.

D. The treatment approach depends on identifying and integrating several factors: the intensity, frequency, and constancy of the symptoms, the nature of the physiological disturbances (i. e. diarrhea or constipation), the degree of psychosocial difficulties, and the frequency of health care utilization.

E. Dietary changes, medications, and psychotherapy can help prevent IBS.

6. Read the introduction in the box and finish the exercises after it.

> *Comparison* is a rhetorical strategy and method of organization in which a writer examines similarities between two people, places, ideas or things. Comparison is also an evaluative tool. In casual use, we often use the terms such as **both**, **similarly**, **likewise** and so on.

1) Circle the compared items and underline the comparative words or phrases.

   Because inflammatory bowel disease (IBD) and irritable bowel syndrome (IBS) are both long-term conditions that affect your gut, they have some similar symptoms such as belly pain, bloating, diarrhea or constipation and defecating more often or feeling like you need to go right away. Both also tend to be diagnosed in young people.

2) Reorder the following sentences to make an effective paragraph.

   A. Both conditions cause inflammation in the stomach lining, but gastritis is general inflammation while an ulcer is a patch of inflamed stomach lining.

   B. Gastritis and stomach ulcers are conditions that affect the small intestine and the stomach.

   C. Ulcers cause more severe, localized pain with the risk of cancer, bleeding, and stomach perforation.

   D. They share many symptoms, such as nausea, vomiting, weight loss, abdominal pain, and loss of appetite.

   E. There are also many differences between the two conditions.

Answer: __ __ __ __ __

7. Translate the Chinese paragraph below into English.

　　肠易激综合征是一种功能性胃肠道疾病,其临床症状包括腹痛、腹胀、排便习惯或大便性状改变。该病与心理因素密切相关,状态焦虑和抑郁的患者,症状容易复发或加重。治疗方法取决于症状的强度、频率和持续性,以及生理紊乱的性质。预防措施包括改变饮食习惯和生活方式、避免紧张的情况,以及使用药物。

8. Read the text and fill in the sheet with proper information.

Reading Prompts	
Items	**Your Answers**
1) *Identify the medical terms concerning **IBS** and group them according to your understanding.*	
2) *Identify the **prepositions** used in "**Epidemiology**"* and expain what conditions they describe.	
3) Identify the **noun phrases** used in "**Diagnosis**" and describe the evaluation procedures.	
4) *Identify the **conjunctions** used in "**Quality of Life**" and point out the logical relation each of them indicates.*	
5) *Identify the **typical sentence patterns**. (**the whole article**)*	
6) *Identify the **topic sentence** and the **supporting sentences** in paragraph 3 in "**Mechanismus/ Pathophysiology**".*	

Title: _____

Eating and food are important to people. Even when we are not actually consuming food, thinking about food and longing for food play a key role in our lives. People have evolved to like eating because it is significant for survival. In addition to its biological function, eating is also a principal social and cultural activity that people tend to enjoy for aesthetic or communal reasons. However, food is no longer a sole source of pleasure and enjoyment nowadays, but has increasingly become a cause of concern because of its potential consequences for ill health. The prime reason for such concern has been the growing epidemic of being overweight resulting from our obesogenic environment with plenty of cheap and high caloric foods available at any place any time. The epidemic of being overweight has spurred research into the health consequences of overeating and overweight.

A healthy diet can be defined as a pattern of food intake that has beneficial effects on health or at least no harmful effects. Although it has proven difficult to specify the exact nutritional elements that contribute to health, there is consensus about the essential features of nutritionally poor-quality diets. These are characterized by higher intakes of processed foods, sugar-sweetened beverages, trans- and saturated fats, and added salt and sugar, and lower intakes of fresh fruits, vegetables, nuts and whole grains. However, as it has proven difficult to establish a firm body of empirical evidence about the specific elements of a healthy diet, governmental expert panels who are responsible for communication of nutritional guidelines to the public tend to derive recommendations from observational studies.

What then does advice for a healthy diet generally entail? Many countries have installed official dietary guidelines, which generally call for a varied and balanced diet that is high in vegetables and fruits, and low in fat, sugar and salt. Healthy diets are also rich in polyunsaturated fatty acid, whole grains and fiber, low-fat or non-fat dairy, fish, legumes, and nuts and low in refined grains, and saturated fatty acids.

In view of the complex information about healthy diet that is released by professional and governmental bodies, the public understanding of healthy nutrition is remarkably accurate and reflects the headlines of dietary guidelines. In a survey amongst 14,331 European consumers, balance and variety, low fat, more fruit and vegetables, and fresh foods were the most mentioned aspects of a healthy diet. Similar findings were reported in a review of 38 international studies, naming vegetables and fruit, less meat, low levels of fat, salt and sugar, and balance, variety and moderation as essential elements of a healthy diet by many consumers.

In recent years, research on nutrition and health has shifted towards a greater emphasis on dietary patterns instead of single nutrients or foods, acknowledging that individuals eat foods in a variety of combinations that may have interactive and potentially cumulative effects on health status. After all, why would the prototypical "apple a day" protect your health if you consume lots of fried foods in the evening?

In contrast with the mixed and inconclusive findings on the effects of specific dietary elements on health (with the exception of the Mediterranean diet), the health effects of overweight and obesity—and thus of eating too much rather than eating a specific diet are relatively straightforward and robust. This corresponds with the results from a systematic review of the association between healthy dietary patterns and weight status, suggesting that quantity of intake plays an important role in weight gain. Being overweight results from eating too much in combination with low levels of physical activity: when energy intake exceeds energy expenditure, the excess energy is stored in the body as fat mass and when fat accumulation is excessive, a person becomes overweight or obesity. Obesity harms virtually every aspect of health, from shortening life and contributing to chronic conditions such as diabetes and cardiovascular disease to interfering with breathing and mood.

There is poor evidence for health protective effects of single foods or nutrients. Only comprehensive dietary patterns such as the Mediterranean diet have been suggested to have quantifiable beneficial effects on health. Moreover, direct health effects of specific nutrients and foods may be negligible when compared with the pervasive health effects of being overweight that is the result of overeating on all kinds of (primarily high caloric) foods.

While good health is important to people, more attention should be paid to how health considerations may actually backfire and make it more difficult for people to change their diet. Possessing correct and useful knowledge of what constitutes a healthy diet seems important, as it is necessary for allowing people to make the "right" choices. It is also important to realize that the core components of healthy diet are still unclear which makes communicating recommendations for healthy diet to the general public quite complex. It is obvious that insight into the health benefits or health risks of specific nutrients, foods, or dietary patterns is beyond the task of health psychologists. Nevertheless, a better insight into valid, reliable and robust nutritional recommendations is mandatory for improving the understanding of the role of behavior in healthy diet.

(Extracted from https://www.tandfonline.com)

Exercises

1. Read the article and write a possible title for it.

2. Answer the following questions according to the passage.

1) What roles does eating play in human society?

2) Why does being overweight become the focus of research?

3) What is a healthy diet?

4) What is an unhealthy diet?

5) What kind of eating habits do you consider to be healthy?

UNIT 12   Ophthalmology

Ophthalmology is a branch of medicine that contains the diagnosis and treatment of eye disorders. At present, uncorrected refractive error, cataract, age-related macular degeneration, glaucoma, and diabetic retinopathy are the leading causes of vision impairment globally.

Part I   Intensive Reading

Myopia

Myopia, also known as short-sightedness or near-sightedness, is an eye disorder where light focuses in front of, instead of on the retina. It is often regarded as a benign disorder, because vision can be corrected with glasses, contact lenses and refractive surgery. Nevertheless, myopia has emerged as a major public health concern for many reasons. It is urgent to call for adequate diagnosis and correction of myopic refractive errors, effective treatment of myopic pathologies, and above all, prevention of myopia.

Epidemiology

East Asia has been faced with an increasing prevalence of myopia and the same trend has been shown in other parts of the world to a lesser extent. In population-based studies on children, the prevalence of myopia varies highly between East Asian populations and other clusters, with generally lower prevalence in rural areas than in urban areas. These geographic and/or ethnic differences can be explained by genetic and/or environmental factors, as evidenced by studies on migrant populations. On the other hand, these differences are not pronounced in adult populations. High myopia may be associated with several ocular complications later in life and can be one of the main causes of visual impairment. In general, the risk of pathologic myopia (PM) increases with the severity of high myopia and age. The prevalence of visual impairment attributed to PM is 7% in western populations and 12%–27% in Asian populations. Studies have reported 25% of high myopia may develop PM; while 50% of those with PM may develop visual impairment as older adults. Based on the current prevalence of high myopia in young adults (6.7%–21.6%) in East Asian countries, the prevalence of visual impairment attributed to PM may increase in the future, as these young adults get older.

Mechanisms/Pathophysiology

Myopia is a common refractive error, characterized by an excessive increase in axial length relative to the refractive power of the eye. The mechanisms of the development of myopia may result from a couple of factors.

- Emmetropization and normal ocular growth in human eyes

When incident parallel rays of light from distant objects are brought to a focus upon the retina without accommodation, it is known as emmetropia. During postnatal eye growth, the precise matching of the axial length (the distance from the anterior corneal surface to the retina along the visual axis) and the optical power of the eye brings the eye to emmetropia. This active regulatory process that harmonizes the expansion of the eye with the optical power of the cornea and the crystalline lens is known as emmetropization. Any disruption to these highly coordinated ocular changes results in the development of refractive errors, wherein distant images are focused either behind (hyperopia) or in front (myopia) of the retina.

- Ocular biometric changes in human myopia

The axial length of the eye is the primary biometric determinant of refractive error; however, the dimensions, curvature, and refractive index of each individual ocular structure contribute to the final refractive state. Ocular biometrics vary considerably throughout childhood, during the development and progression of myopia, and in response to clinical myopia control interventions.

- Other visual cues for emmetropization

Whilst the clarity of the retinal image dominates the nature of ocular growth, other visual cues (e. g. aberrations, accommodation and circadian rhythms) may also influence the process of emmetropization.

- Genetic risk factors for myopia

One key indicator of a genetic basis is familial clustering. In the case of myopia, sibling risk ratios are generally high and even higher for high myopia. Children with myopic parents have a higher prevalence of myopia. The risk of myopia is also high for monozygotic and dizygotic twins.

- Environmental factors on myopia

Myopia represents a "complex" disorder with both environmental and genetic origins. The environmental factors (e. g. light exposure, urbanization, near work, and education) could also affect normal ocular growth and lead to the development of refractive errors.

Diagnosis

Clinical presentation. Myopia is the state of refraction in which parallel rays of light are brought to focus in front of the retina of a resting eye. Myopia is measured by the spherical power in diopters of the diverging lens needed to focus light onto the retina, which can be expressed as the spherical equivalent or refraction in the least myopic meridian. The clinical correlates of myopia include blurred distance vision, eye rubbing and squinting.

Types of myopia. Myopia has been classified as either physiologic or pathologic. Physiologic myopia occurs due to an increase in the axial diameter of the eye over that which is attained by normal growth. Pathologic myopia is caused by an abnormal lengthening of the eyeball and is often associated with thinning of the scleral wall.

Another classification is based on age of onset. Congenital or infantile myopia occurs at birth with a reported prevalence in the full-term newborn varying from 0. 0 to 24. 2 percent. This variability is due to technical difficulties in measuring refraction in newborns. School myopia occurs at approximately 7 – 17 years of age and stabilizes by the late teens or early twenties. Both school and adult-onset myopia are mainly the result of idiopathic causes, while congenital myopia is often associated with other abnormalities.

Severe myopia may be associated with myopic macular degeneration, cataract, glaucoma, peripheral retinal changes (such as lattice degeneration), retinal holes and tears, as well as retinal detachment. Methods of correction of myopia are not without complications including corneal infections due to contact lens wear, corneal scarring or persistent corneal haze from refractive surgery.

Testing for myopia may use several procedures to measure how the eyes focus light and to determine the power of any optical lenses needed to correct the reduced vision. As part of the testing, the person will identify letters on a distance chart. The top number of the fraction is the standard distance at which testing is performed (20 feet). The bottom number is the smallest letter size read.

Using an instrument called a phoropter, a doctor of optometry places a series of lenses in front of the eyes and measures how they focus light using a handheld lighted instrument called a retinoscope. Or the doctor may choose to use an automated instrument that evaluates the focusing power of the eye. The power is then refined based on your responses to determine the lenses that allow the clearest vision. The doctor can conduct this testing without using eye drops to determine how the eyes respond under normal seeing conditions.

In some cases, such as for patients who cannot respond verbally or when some of the eye's focusing power may be hidden, a doctor may use eye drops. The eye drops temporarily keep the eyes from changing focus during testing. Using the information from these tests, along with the results of other tests of eye focusing and eye teaming, the doctor can determine if the person has myopia. He or she will also determine the power of any lens correction needed to provide a clearer vision. Once testing is complete, the doctor can discuss treatment options.

Management

Although an outright cure for nearsightedness has not been discovered, the eye doctor can now offer a number of treatments that may be able to slow the progression of myopia. They include the following methods.

Eyeglasses. For most people with myopia, eyeglasses are the primary choice for correction. Depending on the amount of myopia, you may only need to wear glasses for certain activities like watching a movie or driving a car.

Contact lenses. For some individuals, contact lenses offer clearer vision and a wider field of view than eyeglasses. However, since contact lenses are worn directly on the eyes, they require proper evaluation and care to safeguard eye health.

Ortho-k or CRT. Another option for treating myopia is orthokeratology (ortho-k), also known as corneal refractive therapy (CRT). In this nonsurgical procedure, the patients wear a series of specially designed rigid contact lenses to gradually reshape the curvature of cornea, the front outer surface of the eye. The lenses place pressure on the cornea to flatten it.

Laser procedures. Laser procedures such as LASIK (laser-assisted in-situ keratomileusis) or PRK (photorefractive keratectomy) are also possible treatment options for myopia in adults. A laser beam of light reshapes the cornea by removing a small amount of corneal tissue. The amount of myopia that PRK or LASIK can correct is limited by the amount of corneal tissue that can be safely removed.

Other refractive surgery procedures. People who are highly nearsighted or whose corneas are too thin for laser procedures may be able to have their myopia surgically corrected. A doctor may be able to implant small lenses with the desired optical correction in their eyes. The implant can be placed just in front of the natural lens (phakic intraocular lens implant), or the implant can replace the natural lens (clear lens extraction with intraocular lens implantation). This clear lens extraction procedure is similar to cataract surgery but occurs before a cataract is present.

Quality of Life

Uncorrected refractive error can lead to problems in a person's quality of life related to vision and makes it difficult for them to do tasks pertinent to it. Compared with low and moderate myopia, patients with a high degree of myopia experience impaired quality of life similar to that of patients with keratoconus.

While spectacles and contact lenses are usually the first selection of correcting the refractive error for myopic persons, in the last decade, refractive surgery has found its own advocates even among persons who have worn contact lenses. It is now the most common optional surgery in the world. The quality of life of the myopic subjects who had undergone the refractive surgery is better than those who had worn spectacles or contact lenses. Although the quality of life of the person who had undergone refractive surgery was lower than that of emmetropes, refractive surgery leads to an improvement in the quality of life of myopic subjects.

Prevention

Interventions to control myopia are of two kinds. Those aimed at prevention of myopia need to be minimally invasive since they would be applied to children who do not require glasses.

Outdoor interventions. A cautionary note is that elevated sunshine exposures are associated with a higher incidence of skin cancer, but if the causal factor in myopia protection is visible light rather than ultra violet, as the evidence suggests, then myopia-prevention interventions will probably be compatible with avoidance of ultra violet exposures.

Optical intervention. Optical interventions have been extensively used to slow the progress of myopia. The first optical interventions were based on the idea that myopia was caused by excessive accommodation. Extensive testing of simple corrections and bifocals has given little support to this approach. More recent approaches have been based on achieving more accurate image focus and later interventions have made use of more complex lens designs including progressive addition lenses. The most recent optical devices have been based on the possible role of relative peripheral hyperopia in the development of myopia.

(Extracted from https://eyewiki.aao.org)

Vocabulary

refractive	[rɪ'fræktɪv]	*adj.* 屈光
retinopathy	[retɪ'nɒpəθɪ]	*n.* 视网膜病
corneal	['kɔːnɪəl]	*adj.* 角膜的
retina	['retɪnə]	*n.* 视网膜
postnatal	[ˌpəʊst'neɪtl]	*adj.* 出生后的；初生婴儿的
emmetropia	[ˌemə'trəʊpɪə]	*n.* 屈光正常；正视眼
hyperopia	[ˌhaɪpə'rəʊpɪə]	*n.* 远视
spherical	['sferɪkl]	*adj.* 球状的
monozygotic	[ˌmɒnəʊzaɪ'gɒtɪk]	*adj.* 同卵（的）
dizygotic	[ˌdaɪzaɪ'gɒtɪk]	*adj.* 异卵的
diopter	[daɪ'ɒptə(r)]	*n.* （透镜的）屈光度
diverge	[daɪ'vɜːdʒ]	v. 发散；分岔；分开
meridian	[mə'rɪdɪən]	*n.* 子午线；经线
squint	[skwɪnt]	*n.* 斜视
scleral	[sk'lerəl]	*adj.* 巩膜的
congenital	[kən'dʒenɪtl]	*adj.* 先天的；天生的
macular	['mækjʊlə(r)]	*adj.* 斑点的；（眼球）黄斑的
glaucoma	[glɔː'kəʊmə]	*n.* 青光眼
peripheral	[pə'rɪfərəl]	*adj.* 周围的；外围（的）
lattice	['lætɪs]	*n.* 格栅；斜条结构
optometry	[ɒp'tɒmətrɪ]	*n.* 验光；视力测定
retinoscope	['retənəˌskəʊp]	*n.* 视网膜镜
curvature	['kɜːvətʃər]	*n.* 曲率；弯曲；曲度
intraocular	[ˌɪntrə'ɒkjʊlə(r)]	*adj.* 眼内的
bifocals	[ˌbaɪ'fəʊklz]	*n.* 双光眼镜

Exercises

1. Read the text and explain the following medical phrases.

1) Refractive error

2) Pathologic myopia

3) School myopia

4) Visual cues for emmetropization

5) Optical intervention

2. Answer the following questions according to the text.

1) What are the genetic risk factors for myopia?

2) How is myopia classified?

3) What options are available for myopic people to regain clear vision?

4) Are outdoor interventions effective for myopia? If so, explain the reason.

3. Fill in the blanks with the proper forms of the given words.

distribute	refract	optical	myopia	shape
error	cornea	axial	photoreceptor	chamber

Refractive status is a complex variable, determined by the balance of the optical power of the (1)_____ and the lens and the axial length of the eye. Myopia usually results from an eye that has become too long, particularly through elongation of the vitreal (2)_____. Most children are born hyperopic, with a normal distribution of refractive (3)_____. During the first year or two after birth, the (4)_____ narrows with a mean in the hyperopic range of $+1 - +2$ dioptres (D). This change indicates that there is an active process (5)_____ the distribution of refraction, known as emmetropization. After that period, the cornea stabilizes, but (6)_____ can become more myopic as axial length can continue to increase for another two decades. (7)_____ length is the most variable factor during development, with the strongest correlation with refractive status, with longer eyes more likely to be (8)_____ than shorter eyes. Control of the axial elongation of the eye during development is thus crucial for achieving normal vision. Although axial length is important biologically, refractive error is the clinically meaningful value. (9)_____ correction with spectacles and contact lenses does not change axial length, but alters the optics of vision by making the parallel rays of distant objects diverge, bringing them into focus on the (10)_____ using the natural optics of the eye.

4. **Study the bold-faced words in each of the following sentences and imitate the particular way of writing.**

Mentor Sentence：

☆ In morbidly obese patients，bariatric surgery **can be an effective means of** weight loss.

Imitation Sentence：

☆ Parenteral vaccination **can be an effective means of** inducing protective mucosal responses.

1) High myopia **may be associated with** several ocular complications later in life **and can be one of the main causes of** visual impairment.

Answer：_____ **may be associated with** _____

and can be one of the main causes of _____

2) Myopia **is often regarded as** a benign disorder，**because** vision can be corrected with glasses，contact lenses，and refractive surgery.

Answer：_____ **is often regarded as** _____

because _____

3) Physiological myopia **occurs due to** an increase in the axial diameter of the eye over that which is attained by normal growth.

Answer：_____ **occurs due to** _____

_____

4) Myopia-prevention interventions **will probably be compatible with** avoidance of UV exposures.

Answer：_____ **will**

probably be compatible with _____

5. **Match the following statements with the corresponding sections in the text.**

Epidemiology：_____ Management：_____

Mechanisms/Pathophysiology：_____ Quality of Life：_____

Diagnosis：_____ Prevention：_____

A. Myopia，also known as short-sightedness or near-sightedness，is a very common condition that typically starts in childhood.

B. This disorder affects all populations and is reaching epidemic proportions in East Asia，although there are differences in prevalence between countries.

C. Myopia has been classified into two types generally and severe forms of myopia（pathologic myopia）are associated with a risk of other associated ophthalmic problems.

D. Myopia is resulted from several factors including environmental and genetic risk factors.

E. A range of myopia management and control strategies are available that can treat this condition, but it is clear that understanding the factors involved in delaying myopia onset and slowing its progression will be key to reducing the rapid rise in its global prevalence.

F. Refractive error can still lead to problems in a person's quality of life related to vision but optional surgery is now the most common in the world.

G. Improved public health strategies focusing on early detection or prevention combined with additional effective therapeutic interventions to limit myopia progression are also needed.

6. Read the introduction in the box and finish the exercises after it.

> *Contrast means to discuss differences, in which a writer examines differences between two people, places, ideas or things. In casual use, we often use the terms such as **conversely**, **however**, **in contrast**, **unlike** and so on.*

1) Circle the contrasted items and underline the contrasting words or phrases.

Hyperopia is a condition in which an image of a distant object becomes focused behind the retina, making objects up close appear out of focus. Myopia is a condition in which, opposite of hyperopia, an image of a distant object becomes focused in front of the retina, making distant objects appear out of focus. Both conditions can be improved with corrective lenses such as glasses or contacts as well as safe LASIK surgery.

2) Reorder the following sentences to make an effective paragraph.

A. A slightly higher prevalence of astigmatism in girls (1.9%) than in boys (1.5%) was also observed.

B. Hyperopia occurs more frequently in boys (19.6%) than in girls (18.2%).

C. It was found that myopia occurs more frequently in girls (7.4%) than in boys (5.1%).

Answer: __ __ __

7. Translate the Chinese paragraph below into English.

近视眼睛将光聚焦在视网膜前方,这使得近视人群难以看到或者看不清远处物体。由于近视及与近视相关的眼部疾病患病率越来越高,目前许多光学和药理方法被研发出来,用于控制和阻止近视发展。

8. Read the text and fill in the sheet with proper information.

Reading Prompts	
Items	**Your Answers**
1) *Identify the medical terms concerning* ***myopia*** *and group them according to your understanding.*	
2) *Identify the* ***adjectives*** *used in* **"Clinical presentation"** *and explain what conditions they describe.*	
3) *Identify the* ***conjunctions*** *used in* **"Quality of Life"** *and point out the logical relation each of them indicates.*	
4) *Identify the* ***verbs*** *used in* **Exercise 3** *and point out the changes of verb tenses.*	
5) *Identify the* ***typical sentence patterns.*** *(* ***the whole article*** *)*	
6) *Identify the* ***topic sentence*** *and* ***the supporting sentences in paragraph 3 in*** **"Prevention".**	

Title: _____

According to the January 11, 1999 *Newsweek* magazine, reading glasses are one of the most important inventions of the past 2000 years. According to Dr. J. William Rosenthal, " Philosophers, monks, mathematicians, physicists, microscopists, astronomers and chemists all played vital roles in developing this instrument. "

No one really knows about the early history of image magnification. In ancient times, someone noticed that convex-shaped glass magnified images. Sometime between the year 1000 and 1250 crude technology began to develop regarding reading stones (simple magnifiers). English Franciscan Philosopher Roger Bacon, in his *Opus Majus*, noted that letters could be seen better and larger when viewed through less than half a sphere of glass. Bacon's experiments confirmed the principle of the convex (converging) lens, described by Alhazen, "Father of modern optics," an Arabian mathematician, optician and astronomer at Cairo, and even earlier by the Greeks. Bacon recognized that this could assist weak eyes or the vision of aged persons.

Early recorded evidence demonstrates that glasses first appeared in Pisa, Italy about the year 1286. Technically, they were formed from two primitive convex shaped glass/crystal stones. Each was surrounded by a frame and given a handle. These were then connected together through the ends of their handles by a rivet. They were not really an invention per se but instead a bright idea or "adaptation" of something used earlier—the simple glass stone magnifier. Essentially someone took two existing mounted stones and connected them with a rivet. Most likely, this first pair of glasses were invented by a lay person who wanted to keep the process a secret in order to make a profit. Two monks from the St. Catherine's Monastery, Giordano da Rivalto and Alessandro della Spina, provided the earliest documentation to support this fact. On February 23, 1306, Giordano mentioned them by stating in a sermon "it is not yet twenty years since there was found the art of making eyeglasses which make for good vision, one of the best arts and most necessary that the world has. " He coined the word "Occhiale" (eyeglasses) and its use began to spread throughout Italy and Europe. Friar Spina's 1313 obituary notice mentions, "when somebody else was the first to invent eyeglasses and was unwilling to communicate the invention to others, all by himself he made them and good-naturedly shared them with everybody."

It was definitely the city of Florence that by the middle of the fifteenth century led in innovation, production, sale and spread of spectacles within and outside Italy as attested by documents already or soon to be published. Florence was producing in large quantities not only convex lenses for presbyopes, but also concave lenses for myopes. In addition, Florence had become the leading manufacturer of readily available and affordable good-quality spectacles. The large numbers of spectacles circulating in northwest Europe from the fourteenth century were being mass produced in the Low Countries. They were then manufactured in England in the fifteenth century.

Other centers of production like Germany, France and Netherlands began to appear more frequently in the sources only by the sixteenth century, but they never produced anything near the quantity of the Florentine documentation until well into the seventeenth century. In this period, spectacles were both cheap and plentiful. They were not the expensive vision aids of the clergy, the wealthy, and intellectuals, but instead were extensively used by artisans as well. Almost everyone over forty had to have recourse to them without eliminating entirely the need for magnifying lenses and concave mirrors for close work.

The oldest known pictorial representation of eyeglasses is a fresco in the Chapter House of the Dominican Monastery attached to the Basilica of San Niccolò in Treviso. It was painted by Tommaso da Modena in 1352 and shows Cardinal Hugh of Provence wearing a pair of rivet spectacles. What makes this painting interesting is the fact that the cardinal died before glasses were invented but the painter added spectacles to his fresco as a sign of old age and scholarship. The earliest glasses discovered thus far have been an incomplete pair of rivet spectacles found under the floorboards of the nun's choir-stalls during the 1953 renovations to Kloster Wienhausen in northern Germany.

Five hundred years after they had first been invented, spectacles without sides, which had been originally clamped on top of the nose, reappeared around 1840 as the pince-nez. The improved plastics in the early 1900s heralded a new era in frame styling. During the 1930s, sunglasses became especially popular. By 1950, as described by Pierre Marly of France, spectacles had become a fashion accessory in Europe and North America.

Society has been around for about twenty thousand years. Spectacles did not appear until just over seven hundred years ago. Before that time, nearsighted youth endured a world that was clear only to within four to five feet from where they stood. Farsightedness and more specifically presbyopia affected almost everyone. Then, sometime in the last quarter of the thirteenth century, an unknown, an artisan whose name remains lost, made the first spectacles. In 1946, Vasco Ronchi of Florence stated "when it is all summed up, the fact remains that this world has found lenses on its nose without knowing whom to thank."

(Extracted from https: //prezi. com)

Exercises

1. **Read the article and write a possible title for it.**

2. **Answer the following questions according to the passage.**

   1) What did Bacon write about glasses in his *Opus Majus*?

   2) What was the first pair of eyeglasses made of?

   3) Which city was the earliest leading producer of eyeglasses?

   4) What is the story about Cardinal Hugh of Provence and eyeglasses?

   5) What have now led to the huge increase of spectacle-wearing population?

UNIT 13 Oncology

Oncology is the study of cancer. The field of oncology is divided into three main areas: medical, surgical and radiative. Cancer takes place in every part of human body, including but not limited to breast, lung, colon, rectum and prostate. Many cancers stand a chance to be cured if detected early and treated effectively.

Part I Intensive Reading

Breast Cancer

Breast cancer is a disease in which cells in the breast grow out of control. Breast cancer can begin in different parts of the breast. A breast is made up of three main parts: lobules, ducts and connective tissue. The lobules are the glands that produce milk. The ducts are tubes that carry milk to the nipple. The connective tissue (which consists of fibrous and fatty tissue) surrounds and holds everything together. Most breast cancers begin in the ducts or lobules.

Epidemiology

Breast cancer is the most commonly diagnosed cancer among US women, with an estimated 268,600 newly diagnosed women with invasive disease (48,100 cases of ductal carcinoma) in 2019, accounting for approximately 15.2% – 30% of all new cancer cases among women, depending on the data sources. (In men, the 2019 estimate is 2,670 new cases of breast cancer, accounting for $<1\%$ of all new cancer cases among men.) Each year, nearly 42,000 women die of breast cancer, making it the second-leading cause of cancer deaths among US women after lung cancer. The lifetime risk of dying of breast cancer is approximately 2.6%.

Mechanisms/Pathophysiology

Breast cancer is a globally pervasive disease that significantly affects all races and affects both sexes. Cancerous abnormalities of the breast occur in two types of tissue—ductal epithelium and lobular epithelium. Although most breast cancers arise within the ductal epithelium, malignant cells can also originate within lobular (milk-producing) glands. Aberrations of other breast structures, such as sarcomas and lymphomas, are not typically associated with breast cancer, although some proliferative and non-proliferative benign breast conditions can carry a higher risk of breast cancer development.

Diagnosis

- History and physical examination

The clinical history is directed at assessing cancer risk and establishing the presence or absence of symptoms indicative of breast disease. It should include age at menarche, menopausal status, previouspregnancies, and use of oral contraceptives or post-menopausal hormone replacements. It also includes a personal history of breast cancer and age at diagnosis, as well as a history of other cancers treated with radiation. In addition, a family history of breast cancer and/or ovarian cancer in a first-degree relative should be established. Any significant prior breast history should be elucidated including previous breast biopsies. After the estimated risk for breast cancer has been determined, the patient should be assessed for specific symptoms like breast pain, nipple discharge, malaise, bony pain and weight loss.

Physical examination should include a careful visual inspection with the patient sitting upright. Nipple changes, asymmetry and obvious masses should be noted. The skin must be inspected for changes such as: dimpling, erythema or peau d'orange. After careful inspection and with the patient in the sitting position, the cervical, supraclavicular and axillary lymph node basins are palpated for adenopathy. When palpable, the size, number and mobility should be ascertained. Palpation of the breast parenchyma itself is performed with the patient supine and the ipsilateral arm placed over the head. The subareolar (central quadrant) and each quadrant of both breasts is palpated systematically.

- Diagnostic procedures

Procedures commonly used in breast-cancer diagnosis are mammography, ultrasonography, magnetic resonance imaging (MRI) and PET. However, physical examination remains important because a certain proportion (11%) of breast cancers are not seen on mammography.

Mammography remains the most important diagnostic tool in women with breast tissue that is not dense. After menopause, mammography is generally the best method to discover tiny non-palpable lesions. By contrast, ultrasonography is the most effective procedure to diagnose small tumors in women with dense breast and to differentiate solid lesions from cystic lesions.

MRI is mainly used as a problem-solving method after conventional diagnostic procedures. The technique is highly sensitive and mainly used for the screening of high-risk breast cancer-positive patients. It is also useful for identification of primary foci in non-palpable lesions and axillary metastases with no evidence of a primary focus, and for assessment of response to neoadjuvant chemotherapy. Although MRI has good diagnosis accuracy, the rate of false-positive cases is still high and MRI findings cannot be a sole indication for breast surgery.

PET (positron emission tomography) is presently used to discover undetected metastatic foci in any distant organ and can assess the status of axillary nodes in the preoperative staging process. However, PET could fail to identify low-grade lesions and tumors less than 5 mm in size.

Management

Normally surgery, radiation therapy and chemotherapy are used to treat breast cancer.

- Surgery

Breast conservation is currently the most popular treatment because most carcinomas have a restricted size and large primary tumors could be reduced in size by primary chemotherapy. Total removal of the mammary gland is needed for multicentric invasive carcinomas, extensive intraductal carcinomas, inflammatory carcinomas, and large primary carcinomas not reduced enough in size by neoadjuvant chemotherapy. Scleroderma, which would preclude radiation, could be an additional indication. Early breast recurrences or second ipsilateral carcinoma of restricted size can be treated with a second conservative surgery.

Surgeons are advised to undertake mastectomies in the same operative session as reconstruction of the breast. Several options can be chosen, which range from the simple positioning of an expander to the use of musculocutaneous flaps. One method becoming widely used is the skin-sparing mastectomy that conserves an extensive section of skin as well as the more recent skin and nipple-sparing mastectomy that preserves the nipple-areolar complex. Surgery of the axillary nodes now depends on the results of the sentinel lymph-node biopsy—if negative, unneeded axillary dissection can be avoided. Identical 5-year survival rates were recorded in patients with axillary dissection and in those with axillary dissection only if the sentinel lymph-node biopsy had positive results. DCIS (ductal carcinoma in situ) is mainly treated with mammary resection.

- Radiotherapy

Radiation therapy is the use of high-energy X-rays or other particles to destroy cancer cells. Radiation therapy often helps lower the risk of recurrence in the breast. Radiation therapy may be given after or before surgery.

Adjuvant radiation therapy is given after surgery. Most commonly, it is given after a lumpectomy, and sometimes chemotherapy. Patients who have a mastectomy may or may not need radiation therapy depending on the features of the tumor. Radiation therapy may be recommended after mastectomy if a patient has a larger tumor, cancer in the lymph nodes, cancer cells outside of the capsule of the lymph node, or cancer that has grown into the skin or chest wall as well as for other reasons.

Neoadjuvant radiation therapy is radiation therapy given before surgery to shrink a large tumor, which makes it easier to remove. This approach is uncommon and is usually only considered when a tumor cannot be removed with surgery.

- Therapies using medication

Systemic therapy is the use of medication to destroy cancer cells. Medications circulate through the body and therefore can reach cancer cells throughout the body. The types of systemic therapies used for breast cancer include: chemotherapy, hormonal therapy, targeted therapy and immunotherapy.

Chemotherapy is the use of drugs to destroy cancer cells, usually by keeping the cancer cells from growing, dividing and making more cells. It may be given before surgery to shrink a large tumor, make surgery easier, and/or reduce the risk of recurrence, called neoadjuvant chemotherapy. It may also be given after surgery to reduce the risk of recurrence, called adjuvant chemotherapy.

Hormonal therapy, also called endocrine therapy, is an effective treatment for most tumors that test positive for either estrogen or progesterone receptors (called ER positive or PR positive). Hormonal therapies used in breast cancer treatment act as "anti-hormone" or "anti-estrogen" therapies. They block hormone actions or lower hormone levels in the body. Hormonal therapy may also be called endocrine therapy. The endocrine system in the body makes hormones. Hormonal therapy may be given before surgery to shrink a tumor, make surgery easier, and/or lower the risk of recurrence. This is called neoadjuvant hormonal therapy. It may also be given solely after surgery to reduce the risk of recurrence. This is called adjuvant hormonal therapy.

Targeted therapy is a treatment that targets the cancer's specific genes, proteins, or the tissue environment that contributes to cancer growth and survival. These treatments are very focused and work differently than chemotherapy. This type of treatment blocks the growth and spread of cancer cells and limits damage to healthy cells. Not all tumors have the same targets. To find the most effective treatment, the doctor may run tests to identify the genes, proteins and other factors in the tumor. In addition, research studies continue to find out more about specific molecular targets and new treatments directed at them.

Immunotherapy, also called biologic therapy, is designed to boost the body's natural defenses to fight the cancer. It uses materials made either by the body or in a laboratory to improve, target or restore immune system function.

Quality of Life

Survival rates for women with breast cancer have increased significantly over time due to better tests and scans, earlier detection and improved treatment methods. Doctors commonly use five-year survival rates as a way to discuss prognosis. This is because research studies often follow people for five years—it does not mean you will survive for only five years. Compared with other cancers, breast cancer has one of the highest five-year survival rates if diagnosed early. However, patients reported problems with global quality of life, pain, arm symptoms and body image even after 18 months following their treatments. In addition, most of the functional scores did not improve.

Prevention

Research shows that lifestyle changes can decrease the risk of breast cancer, even in women at high risk. To lower the risk, you can follow the following ways.

• Limit alcohol

The more alcohol you drink, the greater your risk of developing breast cancer. The general recommendation—based on research on the effects of alcohol on breast cancer risk—is to limit yourself to no more than one drink a day, as even small amounts increase risk.

- Maintain a healthy weight

If your weight is healthy, work to maintain that weight. If you need to lose weight, ask your doctor about healthy strategies to accomplish this. Reduce the number of calories you eat each day and slowly increase the amount of exercise.

- Be physically active

Physical activity can help you maintain a healthy weight, which helps prevent breast cancer. Most healthy adults should aim for at least 150 minutes a week of moderate aerobic activity or 75 minutes of vigorous aerobic activity weekly, plus strength training at least twice a week.

- Breast-feed

Breast-feeding might play a role in breast cancer prevention. The longer you breast-feed, the greater the protective effect.

- Limit postmenopausal hormone therapy

Combination hormone therapy may increase the risk of breast cancer. Talk with your doctor about the risks and benefits of hormone therapy. You might be able to manage your symptoms with nonhormonal therapies and medications. If you decide that the benefits of short-term hormone therapy outweigh the risks, use the lowest dose that works for you and continue to have your doctor monitor the length of time you are taking hormones.

(Extracted from https://www. ncbi. nlm. nih. gov)

Vocabulary

epithelium	[ˌepɪˈθiːlɪəm]	n. 上皮;上皮细胞
lobular	[ˈlɒbjʊlə(r)]	adj. 有小叶的;有小裂片的
aberration	[ˌæbəˈreɪʃn]	n. 异常
sarcoma	[saːˈkəʊmə]	n. 肉瘤;恶性毒瘤
lymphoma	[lɪmˈfəʊmə]	n. 淋巴瘤
proliferative	[prəˈlɪfəˌreɪtɪv]	adj. 增殖的;增生的
menarche	[meˈnaːkɪ]	n. 初潮
menopausal	[ˌmenəˈpɔːzl]	adj. 绝经期的;更年期的
malaise	[məˈleɪz]	n. 不适
asymmetry	[ˌeɪˈsɪmətrɪ]	n. 不对称
dimpling	[ˈdɪmplɪŋ]	adj. 坑坑洼洼
erythema	[ˌerɪˈθiːmə]	n. 红斑;红疹
cervical	[səˈvɪkəl]	adj. 颈部的

palpate	[pæl'peɪt]	v. 触诊
adenopathy	[ˌædɪ'nɒpəθɪ]	n. 淋巴结肿大
subareolar	[sʌbeə'rɪələ]	adj. 乳晕下的
mammography	[mæ'mɒɡrəfɪ]	n. 乳房 X 线照相术
metastases	[mə'tæstəsiːz]	n. 转移
axillary	['æksɪlərɪ]	adj. 腋窝的
scleroderma	[ˌsklɪərə'dɜːmə]	n. 硬皮病
ipsilateral	[ˌɪpsɪ'læt(ə)r(ə)l]	adj. 身体同侧的
mastectomy	[mæ'stektəmɪ]	n. 乳房切除术
sentinel	['sentɪnl]	n. 前哨
lumpectomy	[lʌm'pektəmɪ]	n. 乳房肿瘤切除术

Exercises

1. Read the text and explain the following medical phrases.

1) Two tissues in which breast cancer usually occurs

2) Procedures commonly used in breast-cancer diagnosis

3) Treatment strategies for breast cancer

4) Systemic therapies used for breast cancer

2. Answer the following questions according to the text.

1) Why is breast cancer the second leading cause of death among US women?

2) Why is MRI used in clinics?

3) When might a doctor recommend radiation therapy?

4) Do you know how to prevent breast cancer?

3. Fill in the blanks with the proper forms of the given words.

| hormon | duct | mutation | ovarian | mass |
| gene | glandular | abnormal | metastasize | accumulate |

Doctors know that breast cancer occurs when some breast cells begin to grow 1)_____ . These cells divide more rapidly than healthy cells do and continue to 2)_____ , forming a lump or 3)_____ . Cells may 4)_____ through breast to lymph nodes or to other parts of the body. Breast cancer most often begins with cells in the milk-producing 5)_____ (invasive ductal carcinoma). Breast cancer may also begin in the 6)_____ tissue called lobules (invasive lobular carcinoma) or in other cells or tissue within the breast. Doctors estimate that about 5 to 10 percent of breast cancers are linked to gene 7)_____ passed through generations of a family. A number of inherited mutated genes that can increase the likelihood of breast cancer have been identified. The most well-known are breast cancer gene 1 (BRCA1) and breast cancer gene 2 (BRCA2), both of which significantly increase the risk of both breast and 8) _____ cancer. Researchers have identified 9) _____ , lifestyle and environmental factors that may increase the risk of breast cancer. It's not clear why some people who have no risk factors develop cancer, yet other people with risk factors never do. It's likely that breast cancer is caused by a complex interaction of the 10) _____ makeup and the environment.

4. **Study the bold-faced words in each of the following sentences and imitate the particular way of writing.**

Mentor Sentence:

☆ In morbidly obese patients, bariatric surgery **can be an effective means of** weight loss.

Imitation Sentence:

☆ Parenteral vaccination **can be an effective means of** inducing protective mucosal responses.

1) Each year, nearly 42,000 women **die of** breast cancer, **making it the** second-**leading cause of cancer deaths among** US women after lung cancer.

Answer: _____ **die of** _____ ,
making it the _____ **-leading cause of among** _____

_____

2) MRI **is mainly used as** a problem-solving method after conventional diagnostic procedures.

Answer: _____ **is mainly used as** _____

_____

3) Chemotherapy **is the use of** drugs **to** destroy cancer cells, **usually by** keeping the cancer cells from growing, dividing, and making more cells.

Answer: _____ **is the use of** _____ **to** _____ ,
usually by _____

_____

4) Breast conservation **is currently the most popular treatment because** most carcinomas have a restricted size and large primary tumors could be reduced in size by primary chemotherapy.

Answer: _____ **is currently the most popular treatment because** _____

_____

5. Match the following statements with the corresponding sections in the text.

Epidemiology:_____   Management:_____

Mechanisms/Pathophysiology: _____   Quality of Life:_____

Diagnosis:_____   Prevention:_____

A. Breast cancer treatment depends on several factors and can include combinations of surgery, chemotherapy, radiation, hormone and targeted therapy.

B. Breast cancer is a malignant tumor that starts in the cells of the breast.

C. Mammography remains the mainstay breast cancer screening and detection tool but magnetic resonance imaging and ultrasound have become useful diagnostic adjuncts in selecting patient populations.

D. Breast cancer is the most commonly diagnosed cancer among US women with an estimated 268,600 newly diagnosed women with invasive disease in 2019.

E. Breast cancer prevention starts with healthy habits—such as limiting alcohol and staying physically active.

F. Survival rates for women with breast cancer have increased significantly over time due to better tests and scans, earlier detection and improved treatment methods.

6. Read the introduction in the box and finish the exercises after it.

> ***Problem-solution pattern*** *is useful in dividing and arranging the information into two main sections: one will describe the problem and the other the solution. The problem-solving organizational pattern is generally best for persuasive writing, where the general purpose of sharing information is to convince the reader to support a specific course of action.*

1) Circle the problem and underline the solution.

There is no sure way to prevent breast cancer. Nevertheless, there are things one can do that might lower the risk. Many risk factors are beyond control, such as being born female and getting older. However, other risk factors can be changed and may lower the risk. For women who are known to be at increased risk for breast cancer, there are additional steps that might reduce the risk of developing breast cancer. For all women, keep the following three guidelines: a) get to and stay at a healthy weight, b) be physically active and c) avoid or limit alcohol. For women at increased risk of breast cancer, consider the following ways: a) genetic counseling and testing for breast cancer risk (if it has not been done already), b) close observation to look for early signs of breast cancer, c) medicines to lower breast cancer risk and d) preventive (prophylactic) surgery.

2) Reorder the following sentences to make an effective paragraph.

A. It can be given after surgery (known as adjuvant treatment) or in conjunction with chemotherapy prior to surgery (neoadjuvant therapy) to shrink the tumor.

B. Therapy with radiation is often used in addition to surgery and chemotherapy to reduce the chances of the cancer recurring.

C. Radiotherapy can also be used without surgery in patients with advanced metastatic breast cancer to help alleviate symptoms.

Answer：__ __ __

7. **Translate the Chinese paragraph below into English.**

乳腺癌是发生于乳腺上皮或导管上皮的恶性肿瘤,病因尚不完全清楚,可能与家族史和乳腺癌相关基因、生殖因素、性激素、营养与饮食、环境因素等有关。早期乳腺癌大多无明显症状,多在健康普查中发现。大多数乳腺癌是无痛性肿块,晚期出现乳头回缩、乳腺皮肤呈"酒窝症"或橘皮样变、腋窝淋巴结肿大等表现。

8. **Read the text and fill in the sheet with proper information.**

Reading Prompts	
Items	**Your Answers**
1) *Identify the medical terms concerning **breast cancer** and group them according to your understanding.*	
2) *Identify the **adverbs** used in "**Epidemiology**" and "**Mechanisms/Pathophysiology**" and explain what conditions they describe.*	
3) *Identify the **conjunctions** used in "**Diagnosis**" and point out the logical relation each of them indicates.*	

continued

Reading Prompts	
Items	**Your Answers**
4) *Identify the* **verbs** *used in* "**Surgery**" **and** "**Radiotherapy**" *and point out the changes of verb tenses.*	
5) *Identify the* **typical sentence patterns.** (*the whole article*)	
6) *Identify the* **topic sentence** *and the* **supporting sentences in paragraph 3 in** "*Diagnostic procedures*".	

Part II   Extensive Reading

Title: _____

From prehistory to ancient Egypt

Cancer has afflicted humanity from pre-historic times though its prevalence has markedly increased in recent decades in unison with rapidly aging populations and, in the last half century, the increasing risky health behavior in the general population and the increased presence of carcinogens in the environment and in consumer products. The oldest credible evidence of cancer in mammals consists of tumor masses found in fossilized dinosaurs and human bones from prehistoric times. The earliest written record generally regarded as describing human cancer appeared in ancient Egyptian manuscripts discovered in the 19th century, especially the Edwin Smith and George Ebers papyri that has described surgical, pharmacological, and magical treatments. The oldest scientifically documented case of disseminated cancer was that of a 40- to 50-year-old Scythian king who lived in the steppes of Southern Siberia 2,700 years ago. Modern microscopic and proteomic techniques confirmed the cancerous nature of his disseminated skeletal lesions and their prostatic origin.

From ancient Egypt to Greece and Rome

Following the decline of Egypt and Greece, Roman medicine became preeminent, especially with Hippocrates of Kos (460 – c. 370 BCE), and Claudius Galenus (129 – c. 216). Writings attributed to them, describing life-long experiences and observations, became the foundation and repository of medical knowledge for the ensuing 1,500 years.

From Rome to the Middle Ages

With the collapse of Greco-Roman civilization after the fall of Rome in 476 CE, medical knowledge in the Western Roman Empire stagnated and many ancient medical writings were lost. Nevertheless, prominent physician-scholars emerged during the Eastern Roman (Byzantine) Empire including Oribasius of Pergamum (c. 320 – c. 403), Aëtius of Amida (502 – 575), and Paulus Aegineta (625? – 690?) all of whom viewed Galen as the source of all medical knowledge.

From the Middle Ages to World War II

In the early-Renaissance period, progress was made in surgical techniques and treatment of wounds, thanks to the Ambroise Paré (1510 – 1590), surgeon to the French Armies and private physician to three French Kings and the father of modern surgery and forensic pathology. However, this burst of Renaissance knowledge did not extend to cancer. How did cancer begin and what were its causes remained puzzles and several academic institutions promoted the search for an answer. During the early part of the 20th century, the introduction of innovative research tools enabled medical investigators to systematically explore old and new hypotheses on the origin and nature of cancer, leading to incremental progress on many fronts. However, the first reports demonstrating the efficacy of an anticancer drug in humans, albeit modest, took place towards the end of World War II. Ironically, that drug was derived from mustard gas, a blistering agent first introduced as a chemical warfare agent by the Imperial German Army but widely used in World War I by both Germany and the Allies. While surgery is most adept and successful at managing early stage cancer, today's treatment of inoperable cancer relies on a variety of agents administered orally or intravenously with or without surgery, radiotherapy or biological agents as adjuvants. Cancer chemotherapy is a recent development with its historical origins in observations of the toxic effects of mustard gas (sulfur mustard) in World War I.

Evolution of cancer treatments: immunotherapy

Better understanding of the biology of cancer cells has led to the development of biologic agents. Clinical trials have shown that this cancer treatment, called biological response modifier therapy, biologic therapy, biotherapy or immunotherapy is effective for many types of cancer. Scientists are also studying vaccines that boost the body's immune response to cancer cells.

Evolution of cancer treatments: targeted therapy

Until the late 1990s nearly all drugs used in cancer treatment (with the exception of hormone treatments) worked by killing cells that were in the process of replicating their DNA and dividing to form new cells. Targeted therapies work by influencing the processes that control growth, division, and spread of cancer cells, as well as the signals that cause cancer cells to die naturally.

Advancement of cancer survivorship

Because more people are surviving cancer, behavioral researchers are working to learn more about the problems that survivors face. Some of these problems are permanent side effects of treatment, the possibility of second cancers caused by treatment, and emotional or social challenges, like getting health insurance and discrimination by employers. Cancer was once a word that people were afraid to speak in public. Now, the view that cancer cannot be cured is slowly changing.

Cancer in the twenty-first century

Cancer research is advancing on so many fronts that it's hard to choose the ones to highlight, but here are a few examples:

Immunotherapy. Drugs aimed at specific immune checkpoints are being developed to help the immune system better kill cancer cells.

More on cancer genetics. Researchers are looking for gene mutations that cause some patients to respond better to certain drugs.

Nanotechnology. New technology for producing materials that form extremely tiny particles is leading to very promising imaging tests that can more accurately show the location of tumors.

Robotic surgery. This term refers to manipulation of surgical instruments remotely by robot arms and other devices controlled by a surgeon.

Expression profiling and proteomics. Expression profiling allows scientists to determine relative output of hundreds or even thousands of molecules (including the proteins made by RNA, DNA, or even a cell or tissue) at one time.

(Extracted from http://www. medicinacomplementar. com. br)

Exercises

1. **Read the article and write a possible title for it.**

2. **Answer the following questions according to the passage.**

   1) When was human cancer first recorded?

   2) Why did medicine in the Western Roman Empire stagnate?

   3) From what was the first-reported anticancer drug derived?

   4) What are the side effects of chemotherapy?

   5) What problems may cancer survivors face?

UNIT 14   Fever

Fever, a common sign of illness, is a temporary increase of body temperature. While countless over-the-counter medications cool down fevers, sometimes it is better left untreated. In fact, fever as an immune means plays a key role in defending infections.

Part I   Intensive Reading

Severe Acute Respiratory Syndrome

The severe acute respiratory syndrome (SARS) is responsible for the first pandemic of the 21st century. Within months after its emergence, it had affected more than 8,000 patients in 26 countries on five continents. It illustrated dramatically the potential of air travel and globalization for the dissemination of an emerging infectious disease and highlighted the need for a coordinated global response to contain such disease threats.

Epidemiology

To date, there have been a few preliminary attempts at modeling that will permit the quantitative assessment of the epidemic potential of SARS and the effectiveness of control measures. The results indicate that the SARS coronavirus is less transmissible than was initially thought, with the average number of secondary cases resulting from each case estimated to be two to four overall. However, one feature of this disease is that a few infected persons have been responsible for a disproportionate number of transmissions—the so-called super-spreading events. These results suggest that SARS coronavirus is sufficiently transmissible to cause a very large epidemic if it is left unchecked but that it is not so contagious overall as to be uncontrollable with good basic public health measures.

Most studies of SARS cases in which transmission occurred from a single point of exposure estimated the incubation period to be between 2 and 10 days with a median ranging from 4 to 7 days. However, with the application of maximum-likelihood methods, the mean incubation period was calculated to be 6 days, and the maximal incubation period 14 days. Recent studies indicate that some cases may have developed after incubation periods of up to 20 days, although data on the history of exposure were incomplete. However, public health measures based on the maximal incubation period of 10 days, which the World Health Organization (WHO) estimated on the basis of studies, were successful in interrupting the chain of infection globally.

The primary mode of transmission appears to be through direct or indirect contact of mucous membrane (eyes, nose or mouth) with infectious respiratory droplets or fomites. The use of aerosol-generating procedures (such as endotracheal intubation, bronchoscopy and treatment with aerosolized medication) in hospitals may amplify the transmission of SARS coronavirus. The role of fecal-oral transmission is unknown but may be important, given that profuse watery diarrhea is a common feature of the disease and that SARS coronavirus is shed in large quantities in stool.

To date, there have been two reported cases of transmission from children to adults and no reports of transmission from children to other children. There have been no reports of vertical or perinatal transmission. A combination of tracing of contacts and molecular epidemiological data provides a better understanding of the genesis of the SARS pandemic.

The role of seasonality in the transmission of SARS coronavirus is currently unknown. Many respiratory viruses, including the human coronaviruses, are most common in the winter. However, this is not true of all respiratory viruses and all geographic regions.

Mechanisms/Pathophysiology

In general, people at greatest risk of SARS are those who have had close contact with someone who is infected, such as family members and health care workers.

SARS coronavirus is transmitted primarily through droplets entering the human body via the respiratory tract mucosa and causing viremia. Angiotensin-converting enzyme 2 (ACE 2) has been identified as a functional receptor for SARS coronavirus. The incubation period is 2 to 10 days and the risk of transmission is greater during the second week of illness, which correlates with the timing of peak viral load. The possibility of fomite transmission and airborne transmission cannot be excluded although the role of fecal-oral or fecal-respiratory spread seems to be of minor importance. Although each SARS case is expected to infect 2 to 4 people, it is thought that, in the pandemic of 2002 to 2003, a small number of infected individuals were responsible for a disproportionate number of transmissions in so-called super-spreading events, and that it was through this mechanism that the SARS outbreak disseminated globally.

There are 3 phases in the course of the disease: viral replication, inflammatory pneumonitis and pulmonary fibrosis. Pathologic findings of the lungs include diffuse alveolar damage, desquamation of pneumocytes, hyaline membrane formation and inflammatory infiltrates. The longer the course of the disease, the more extensive the fibrous organization of the lung tissue.

Clinical deterioration in some patients during the third week of illness, despite a fall in viral load, suggests that immune dysregulation may play a role. Furthermore, the HLA-B*4601 haplotype has been associated with the severity of SARS infection, suggesting the existence of a genetic predisposition.

Diagnosis

SARS has flu-like symptoms that usually begin 2 to 7 days after infection and its symptoms include:

□ *fever*
□ *fatigue*
□ *headaches*
□ *chills*
□ *muscle pain*
□ *loss of appetite*
□ *diarrhea*

After these symptoms, the infection will begin to affect your lungs and airways (respiratory system), leading to additional symptoms, such as:

□ *a dry cough*
□ *breathing difficulties*
□ *an increasing lack of oxygen in the blood, which can be fatal in the most severe cases*

SARS is a viral pneumonia that progresses rapidly. The initial manifestations of SARS are not specific and it cannot be clinically differentiated from other acute community-acquired pneumonias. The occurrence of lower respiratory disease, particularly pneumonia, in epidemiologically linked clusters of patients raises the level of suspicion but is not unique to SARS. Diseases such as influenza can cause similar outbreaks. The case definition of SARS has been refined over time. Additional cases were uncovered through daily clinical and radiographic follow-up evaluation of epidemiologically linked patients who did not meet a sufficient number of criteria to satisfy the case definition. Given the lack of characteristic clinical features associated with SARS, the definition of cases had to rely heavily on the contact history of known patients.

The RT-PCR tests that were in use during April and May 2003 lacked sensitivity during the first five days of illness but had better sensitivity in later stages of the illness. However, it was demonstrated that respiratory and fecal specimens are suitable for diagnosis with the use of RT-PCR. Although specimens from the lower respiratory tract are the most useful for viral diagnosis, few patients with SARS have a productive cough early in the course of illness. Thus, nasopharyngeal swabs and throat and nose swabs are the primary types of specimens that have been investigated. Viral RNA is also detectable in serum or plasma, as well as in urine. More recently, improved methods of extracting specimens and real-time RT-PCR assays have improved the sensitivity of testing during the first few days of illness and are now the mainstay for early diagnosis.

Management

Although a number of strategies have been used for specific treatment and prevention, controlled studies documenting the efficacy of therapies are lacking. Patients with suspected SARS are initially treated empirically with broad-spectrum antibacterial drugs that are effective against other agents that cause typical and atypical acute community-acquired pneumonia to exclude these diagnoses. Before the causative agent was known, ribavirin was used by some as a broad-spectrum empirical antiviral agent for the treatment of patients with SARS.

Testing for susceptibility to antiviral drugs suggests that interferon beta, glycyrrhizin (licorice-root extract), and to a lesser extent, interferon alfa have activity against SARS coronavirus. In an experimental model of SARS coronavirus infection, treatment both before exposure and after exposure with pegylated interferon alfa reduced viral replication, and preliminary uncontrolled studies of combinations of interferon and corticosteroids in humans suggest that there are no obvious adverse effects.

Randomized, placebo-controlled clinical trials appear to be warranted.

There are a number of potential targets for antiviral drugs in the replication cycle of SARS coronavirus, including fusion inhibitors and protease inhibitors. The availability of the full genome sequence of the virus provides the basis for targeted strategies to develop antiviral drugs and vaccines. Unlike other acute respiratory viral infections, SARS is characterized by a peak in the viral load in respiratory secretions occurring around the 10th day of illness and a subsequent decrease, concomitant with the appearance of an antibody response to the virus. Some patients have deterioration during the second week of illness in spite of a decreasing viral load and it has been suggested that part of the damage to the lungs may be immunopathologic in nature. Some have reported that early therapy with regimens of high-dose methylprednisolone is useful in modulating the damage to the lungs, but no data from randomized, placebo-controlled trials are available to confirm a clinical benefit. Doctors also use a number of other therapeutic options, including thymic peptides or recombinant human thymus proteins, intravenous immunoglobulin, IgM-enriched immunoglobulin, plasma from patients in the convalescent phase, and traditional Chinese medicine.

Patients with unrecognized SARS, especially those with an atypical presentation, the elderly and the chronically ill, have been the source of a number of outbreaks and pose a challenge to infection control in hospitals. Thus, a high index of suspicion is required in the recognition of cryptic cases of SARS and infection-control standards must be reinforced in all parts of the hospital.

Quality of Life

There was a significant impairment in both the quality of life and mental functioning. The exercise capacity and health status of SARS survivors was considerably lower than that of a normal population at 6 months. Significant impairment in surface area for gas exchange was noted in 15.5% of survivors. The functional disability appears out of proportion to the degree of lung function impairment and may be related to additional factors such as muscle deconditioning and steroid myopathy.

The high mortality and social dislocation caused by SARS, and the universal publicity given to it, have resulted in stress, anxiety and vulnerability during the patients' acute illnesses. Patients with SARS were banned from visiting with relatives, some of whom became infected and some of whom died. It also appears that this predominately pulmonary disease has a greater impact on one's physical health than on one's mental health with more profound adverse effects on women because men could probably tolerate more stress in both functional and psychological aspects.

For there are obvious deficits in the cardiopulmonary performance and muscular strength and endurance among SARS patients, some physical rehabilitation programs are needed to improve their physical profiles and quality of life. These patients require a supervised and tailored exercise program, which may boost their physical and emotional performance.

Prevention

In response to the outbreak of Severe Acute Respiratory Syndrome (SARS) in several countries, the World Health Organization has developed the following guidelines to prevent SARS:

□ *Wash your hands often with soap and water for 20 seconds, and help young children do the same.*

□ *Cover your nose and mouth with a tissue when you cough or sneeze, then throw the tissue in the trash.*

□ *Avoid touching your eyes, nose, and mouth with unwashed hands.*

□ *Avoid close contact, such as kissing, or sharing cups or eating utensils, with sick people.*

□ *Clean and disinfect frequently touched surfaces, such as toys and doorknobs.*

(Extracted from *New England Journal of Medicine*)

Vocabulary

aerosol	[ˈerəsɔːl]	n. 气溶胶
angiotensin	[ˌændʒɪəʊˈtensən]	n. 血管紧缩素
convalescent	[ˌkɒnvəˈlesənt]	adj. 恢复期的
desquamation	[ˌdeskwəˈmeɪʃn]	n. 脱屑;脱皮
disproportionate	[ˌdɪsprəˈpɔːrʃənət]	adj. 不成比例的
disseminate	[dɪˈsemɪneɪt]	v. 散播
endotracheal	[ˌendəʊˈtreɪkɪəl]	adj. 气管内的
fibrosis	[faɪˈbrəʊsɪs]	n. 纤维症
glycyrrhizin	[glɪˈkɜːraɪzɪn]	n. 甘草素
haplotype	[ˈhæpləʊtaɪp]	n. 单倍体
hyaline	[ˈhaɪəlɪn]	adj. 透明的
pegylated	[ˈpiːdʒɪleɪtɪd]	adj. 加入聚乙二醇的
peptide	[ˈpeptaɪd]	n. 肽

placebo	[plə'siːbəʊ]	*n.* 安慰剂
recombinant	[ri'kæmbənənt]	*n.* 重组细胞
specimen	['spesɪmən]	*n.* 标本；样本
viremia	[vaɪ'riːmɪə]	*n.* 病毒血症

Exercises

1. Read the text and explain the following medical phrases.

1) Symptoms of SARS

2) Risk factors for SARS

3) The official maximal incubation period of SARS

4) General treatment of SARS

2. Answer the following questions according to the text.

1) What types of individuals are high-risk group of SARS?

2) What tests may a doctor recommend to diagnose SARS?

3) What are the phases in the course of SARS?

4) Do you know how to prevent SARS?

3. Fill in the blanks with the proper forms of the given words.

| bronchoalveolar | necropsy | epidemiology | teleconference | serology |
| routine | initiate | antigenical | transcript | influenza |

On March 18, 2003, WHO 1)＿＿＿＿ a virtual network of laboratories to investigate the cause of SARS. Daily 2) ＿＿＿＿ updated members of the network on the progress of laboratory investigations in different parts of the world on patients with suspected SARS. This investigation established that 3)＿＿＿＿ and other common respiratory pathogens were not the cause of this novel disease syndrome. Strategies for the detection of a novel agent included the use of direct electron microscopy on respiratory specimens, 4) ＿＿＿＿ lavage, and lung tissue obtained from lung biopsy or 5)＿＿＿＿, culture in cell lines known to support respiratory viral infection (and subsequently on other types of cells), PCR and reverse-6) ＿＿＿＿ PCR（RT-PCR）with consensus primers for respiratory viral pathogens, and random-primer RT-PCR. 7)＿＿＿＿ was used to detect agents 8)＿＿＿＿ related to known respiratory pathogens. One of the problems faced in this investigation was the differentiation of SARS from more 9)＿＿＿＿ causes of atypical pneumonia. The one feature supporting the probable diagnosis of SARS was 10)＿＿＿＿ linkage to a cluster of similar disease cases.

4. **Study the bold-faced words in each of the following sentences and imitate the particular way of writing.**

Mentor Sentence:

☆ In morbidly obese patients, bariatric surgery **can be an effective means of** weight loss.

Imitation Sentence:

☆ Parenteral vaccination **can be an effective means of** inducing protective mucosal responses.

1) To date, there have been a few **preliminary attempts at** modeling that will permit the quantitative assessment of the epidemic potential of SARS and the effectiveness of control measures.

Answer: _____ **preliminary attempts at** _____

_____

_____

2) **Clinical deterioration in some patients during** the third week of illness, despite a fall in viral load, **suggests that** immune dysregulation may play a role.

Answer: **Clinical deterioration in some patients during** _____

_____ , **suggests that** _____

_____

3) **Patients with** suspected SARS **are initially treated empirically with** broad-spectrum antibacterial drugs that are effective against other agents that cause typical and atypical acute community-acquired pneumonia to exclude these diagnoses.

Answer: **Patients with** _____ **are initially treated empirically with** _____

4) **Unlike other** acute respiratory viral infections, SARS **is characterized by** a peak in the viral load in respiratory secretions occurring around the 10th day of illness and a subsequent decrease, **concomitant with** the appearance of an antibody response to the virus.

Answer: **Unlike other** _____ , _____ **is characterized by** _____ , **concomitant with** _____

5. **Match the following statements with the corresponding sections in the text.**

Epidemiology: _____   Management: _____

Mechanisms/Pathophysiology: _____   Quality of Life: _____

Diagnosis: _____   Prevention: _____

A. Given the lack of characteristic clinical features associated with SARS, the definition of cases had to rely heavily on the contact history of known patients.

B. This investigation shows a significant impairment in both the QoL and mental functioning.

C. The course of SARS consists of viral replication, inflammatory pneumonitis, and pulmonary fibrosis.

D. There is currently no cure for SARS, but research to find a vaccine is ongoing.

E. Prevention is, so far, the best practice in order to reduce the impact of SARS.

F. SARS has been transmitted primarily, but not exclusively, in health care and hospital settings, generally five or more days after the onset of disease and from patients who were severely ill.

6. **Read the introduction in the box and finish the exercises after it.**

> ***Order of importance***, *widely used in sciences, especially lab texts and experiments, shows information **from** either **the most important part to the least important part** or vice versa. The writer might begin a paragraph with the supporting detail that "packs the most punch" and end with a weaker idea. The writer can also do the opposite by beginning the paragraph with a less forceful idea and ending it with a stronger one.*

1) Circle the most important information and underline the less important ones.

　　After-effects of SARS will be felt for a long time to come, the most painful of which will be on the families of the deceased. The Committee extends its sympathies to those who have lost loved ones as a result of SARS. The disease will also have left an indelible mark on those who suffered from it, their carers, families and friends, and the many individuals who contributed to the fight against SARS, both in the frontline and behind the scenes. Finally, the community as a whole has had to come to terms with the potentially devastating effects of a new and frightening infection.

2) Reorder the following sentences to make an effective paragraph.

　A. In one study, 57% of children had lymphopenia on presentation, and this frequency rose to 91%.

　B. The most striking laboratory finding is absolute lymphopenia.

　C. The mean value was $0.9\pm0.7\times10^{-9}$/L.

　D. Other frequently abnormal laboratory findings include thrombocytopenia and elevated lactate dehydrogenase and creatinine phosphokinase.

　E. This occurs in nearly all pediatric patients.

Answer：__ __ __ __ __

7. **Translate the Chinese paragraph below into English.**

严重急性呼吸综合征简称 SARS,是一种因感染 SARS 型冠状病毒引起的严重急性呼吸道疾病,具有很强的传染性。该病临床表现主要以发热、胸闷、干咳为主,如果不及时控制,可能会迅速导致呼吸系统衰竭,最终危及生命。

8. **Read the text and fill in the sheet with proper information.**

Reading Prompts	
Items	**Your Answers**
1) *Identify the medical terms concerning* **SARS** *and group them according to your understanding.*	
2) *Identify the* **adjectives** *used in* "**Diagnosis**" *and explain what conditions they describe.*	
3) *Identify the* **conjunctions** *used in* "**Epidemiology**" *and point out the logical relation each of them indicates.*	
4) *Identify the* **verbs** *used in* **Exercise 3** *and point out the changes of verb tenses.*	
5) *Identify the* **typical sentence patterns.** (*the whole article*)	
6) *Identify the* **topic sentence** *and the* **supporting sentences in paragraph 1 in** "*Quality of Life*")	

Title: _____

It is no secret that vaccinations have revolutionized global health. Arguably, the single most life-saving innovation in the history of medicine, vaccines have eradicated smallpox, slashed child mortality rates, and prevented lifelong disabilities. Possibly lesser known, however, are the historic events and pioneers we can today thank for not only saving millions of lives each year, but for laying the foundations of future vaccine development.

Early attempts to inoculate people against smallpox—one of history's most feared illnesses, with a death rate of 30%—were reported in China as early as the 16th Century. Smallpox scabs could be ground up and blown into the recipient's nostrils or scratched into their skin. The practice, known as "variolation," came into fashion in Europe in 1721, with the endorsement of English aristocrat Lady Mary Wortley Montagu, but was later met with public outcry after it transpired 2%–3% of people died after inoculation, and further outbreaks were triggered.

The next iteration of inoculation, which turned out to be much safer than variolation, originated from the observation that dairy farmers did not catch smallpox. The 18th Century English physician, Edward Jenner, hypothesized that prior infection with cowpox—a mild illness spread from cattle—might be responsible for the suspected protection against smallpox. Therefore, he set to work on a series of experiments, now considered the birth of immunology, vaccine therapy and preventive health.

In 1796, Jenner inoculated an eight-year-old boy by taking pus from the cowpox lesions on a milkmaid's hands and introducing the fluid into a cut he made in the boy's arm. Six weeks later, Jenner exposed the boy to smallpox, but he did not develop the infection then, or on subsequent exposures. In the years that followed, Jenner collected evidence from a further 23 patients infected or inoculated with the cowpox virus to support his theory that immunity to cowpox did indeed provide protection against smallpox.

The earliest vaccination—the origin of the term coming from the Latin for cow ("vacca")—was born. Jenner's vaccination quickly became the major means of preventing smallpox around the world, even becoming mandatory in some countries.

Almost a century after Jenner developed his technique, in 1885, the French biologist, Louis Pasteur, saved a nine-year-old boy's life after he was bitten by a rabid dog, by injecting him with a weakened form of the rabies virus each day for 13 days. The boy never developed rabies and the treatment was heralded a success. Pasteur coined his therapy a "rabies vaccine", expanding the meaning of vaccine beyond its origin. The global influence of Louis Pasteur led to the expansion of the term vaccine to include a long list of treatments containing live, weakened, or killed viruses, typically given in the form of an injection, to produce immunity against an infectious disease.

Scientific advances in the first half of the 20th century led to an explosion of vaccines that protected against whooping cough (1914), diphtheria (1926), tetanus (1938), influenza (1945) and mumps (1948). Thanks to new manufacturing techniques, vaccine production could be scaled up by the late 1940s, setting global vaccination and disease eradication efforts in motion. Vaccines against polio (1955), measles (1963), rubella (1969) and other viruses were added to the list over the decades that followed, and worldwide vaccination rates shot up dramatically thanks to successful global health campaigns.

By the late 1990s, the progress of international immunization programs was stalling. Nearly 30 million children in developing countries were not fully immunized against deadly diseases and many others were not immunized at all. The problem was that new vaccines were becoming available but developing countries simply could not afford them.

Protecting against long-standing illnesses will continue to be important in the decades and centuries ahead, but the work is not complete. In order to protect the world against infectious diseases, we need a mechanism to monitor new viruses, and rapidly develop vaccines against the most dangerous emerging infections. The devastating Ebola virus was a wake-up call for how ill prepared the world was to handle such an epidemic. A vaccine was eventually approved but came too late for the thousands of people who lost their lives.

In response, the Coalition for Epidemic Preparedness Innovation was launched at Davos in 2017, a global partnership between public, private, philanthropic, and civil society organizations working to accelerate the development of vaccines against emerging infectious diseases and enable equitable access to these vaccines for affected populations during outbreaks.

We have come a long way since the risky and gruesome early inoculation efforts five centuries ago. Scientific innovation, widespread global health campaigns, and new public-private partnerships are literally lifesavers. Finding a vaccine to protect the world against a new virus is an enormous challenge, but if there is one thing we can learn from history, it's that there is reason for hope.

(Extracted from https://www.weforum.org)

Exercises

1. Read the article and write a possible title for it.

2. Answer the following questions according to the passage.

1) What have vaccines contributed to human society?

2) What has Louis Pasteur contributed to vaccination?

3) What diseases had been prevented by vaccination by 1970s?

4) What new challenges may humans face today toward vaccination?

5) How can we fight against new viruses?

UNIT 15 Endocrinology

Endocrinology is a branch of medicine that studies endocrine system, which controls the hormones in the human body. Endocrine diseases are caused when hormone levels are too high or too low, or when the body does not react to hormones the way it is supposed to. Some well-known endocrine disorders are diabetes, hyperthyroidism, hypothyroidism and Cushing's syndrome.

Part I Intensive Reading

Diabetes Mellitus

Diabetes Mellitus (DM) is a metabolic disorder characterized by the presence of chronic hyperglycemia either immune-mediated (type 1 diabetes), insulin resistance (type 2 diabetes), gestational or others (environment, genetic defects, infections, and certain drugs).

Epidemiology

Diabetes remains as the 5th leading cause of death worldwide and has directly resulted in 1.6 million deaths. Diabetic patients are reported to have a 15% increased risk of premature death and life expectancy reduced by approximately 10 and 20 years for type 1 and type 2 diabetes respectively.

By 2030, diabetes is estimated to affect 439 million adults, up from the previous estimation of 366 million. However, statistics show that the number of diabetic patients worldwide was 422 million in 2014. Thus, a new report has estimated that there will be at least 592 million diabetes cases worldwide in 2035.

Diabetes is also reported to be more prevalent in the urban population when compared to the rural population, and affects more men than women. Diabetes can affect anyone, but many studies that date back to as early as 1969 show that Asians, people who origin from the East Asia, Southeast Asia, and particularly South Asia, are more susceptible to diabetes than people from other ethnicities.

Mechanisms/Pathophysiology

There are generally 3 types of diabetes: type 1, 2 and gestational diabetes, but more emphasis is placed on the first two types of diabetes. Currently, although type 1 diabetes cannot be prevented, type 2 is preventable with exercising and healthy diet.

Type 1 diabetes mellitus. Type 1 diabetes is a result of β-cell destruction which customarily provokes complete insulin insufficiency. It was formerly known as insulin-dependent, juvenile or childhood-onset diabetes. It is occasioned by an autoimmune reaction, in which the immune system invaded against the insulin-producing pancreatic beta cells. Type 1 diabetes is distinguished by deficient insulin production in the body. In such type of diabetes mellitus, the patients require daily administration of insulin so as to normalize the glucose level in the blood. Extreme urination and thirst, continuous hunger, weight loss, vision changes and fatigue are the main symptoms of type 1 diabetes.

Type 2 diabetes mellitus. Type 2 diabetes is the most typical diabetes mellitus. Earlier, type 2 diabetes is termed as non-insulin-dependent or adult-onset diabetes. It is caused by a combination of two primary factors: defective insulin secretion by pancreatic β-cells and the inability of insulin-sensitive tissues to respond appropriately to insulin. For many years, type 2 diabetes was observed only in adults; nowadays it has started to be seen also in children.

Gestational diabetes. Gestational diabetes is a type of diabetes determined in the second or third trimester of pregnancy, which is not clearly overt diabetes. It is a provisional disorder that happens in pregnancy and brings enduring danger of type 2 diabetes. Women with slightly elevated blood glucose levels are diagnosed as having gestational diabetes, while women with substantially elevated blood glucose levels are classified as having diabetes mellitus in pregnancy. Screening by means of an oral glucose tolerance test is therefore recommended and must be conducted early in pregnancy for high risk women. Women with hyperglycemia diagnosed during pregnancy are at greater risk of adverse pregnancy outcomes such as very high blood pressure and fetal macrosomia with the vaginal birth being difficult and risky.

Gestational diabetes normally disappears after delivery, but women who have been previously diagnosed are in danger of presenting gestational diabetes in subsequent pregnancies and type 2 diabetes later in their life. In addition, infants borne by mothers with gestational diabetes also have a higher risk of developing type 2 diabetes during adolescence or early adulthood.

Diagnosis

Urine test and blood tests are conducted to detect diabetes by checking for excess body glucose. To be diagnosed as diabetic, one's blood glucose level needs to be equal to or above a certain value. According to the American Diabetes Association (ADA), there are four methods for the diagnosis of diabetes and the same methods are used for the screening of prediabetes in patients. The commonly conducted tests for determining whether a person has diabetes or not are fasting plasma glucose (FPG) test, A1C test, oral glucose tolerance test (OGTT) and random plasma glucose (RPG) test.

Fasting plasma glucose test (FPG). Fasting refers to the absence of food and drink intake, apart from water, for at least 8 hours before the test. A fasting blood glucose level less than 100 mg/dL (5.6 mmol/L) is normal. A fasting blood glucose level from 100 to 125 mg/dL (5.6 to 6.9 mmol/L) is considered prediabetes. Diabetes is diagnosed at fasting blood glucose of greater than or equal to 126 mg/dL (7 mmol/L).

Oral glucose tolerance test (OGTT). In OGTT, patient consumes a glucose syrup solution containing 75 g of glucose before which a blood test is carried out to determine 2 hour plasma glucose (PG). A blood sugar level less than 140 mg/dL (7.8 mmol/L) is normal. A reading of more than 200 mg/dL (11.1 mmol/L) after 2 hours indicates diabetes. A reading between 140 and 199 mg/dL (7.8 mmol/L and 11.0 mmol/L) indicates prediabetes.

Glycated hemoglobin or hemoglobin bounded to glucose (A1C). The A1C test is used to assess glycemic control. The results reflect the average glycemia (glucose concentration) over approximately 3 months. A1C measurements for diagnosis of diabetes should be performed by a clinical laboratory because of the lack of standardization of point-of-care testing. One advantage of using A1C measurement is the ease of testing because it does not require fasting. An A1C between 5.7% and 6.4% indicates prediabete and below 5.7% is considered normal. Diabetes is diagnosed at an A1C of greater than or equal to 6.5%.

Random plasma glucose (RPG) test. Random means that the test can be taken at any time of a day without fasting. A random plasma glucose test result above 200 mg/dL (11.1 mmol/L), paired with symptoms like extreme thirst, hunger, or fatigue, is indicative of diabetes.

Management

- Type 1 diabetes

Self-monitoring. The conventional approach, practiced by approximately 83% of patients with type 1 diabetes, is to monitor glucose levels via capillary blood testing. Testing is advised before meals, before exercise, before bedtime, occasionally postprandially, and anytime hypoglycemia is perceived. The newer practice of continuous glucose monitoring, used by approximately 17% of persons with type 1 diabetes, can also achieve tight glycemic control. Compared with conventional self-monitoring, continuous glucose monitoring has been associated with improved glycemic control. However, the significant increase in cost associated with continuous glucose monitoring needs to be considered when an individual is choosing between glucose monitoring approaches.

Insulin therapy. Patients with type 1 diabetes require lifelong insulin therapy. Consensus guidelines recommend intensive treatment with a combination of multiple mealtime bolus and basal injections or continuous insulin infusion through an insulin pump. Approximately 64% of persons with type 1 diabetes in the United States use an insulin pump. Most patients who use the pump use rapid-acting insulin, e. g. aspart (Novolog), glulisine (Apidra), lispro (Humalog), whereas a small minority still use regular insulin. Choice of insulin type needs to account for duration of action, cost and route of administration.

- Type 2 diabetes

Compared with type 1 diabetes mellitus patients, the majority of type 2 patients typically do not require daily insulin doses. The disease can be treated with oral medications and changes in lifestyle until resistance becomes difficult to control, after which an insulin regimen is usually required.

Lifestyle modification. Certain epigenetic risk factors, such as obesity, lack of physical exercise, and a physically inactive lifestyle worsens the insulin resistance. Lifestyle modification mainly comprises regular and nutritious dietary advice, instructions for physical activities and weight loss. Dietary intake and physical exercise are the two main determinants of the energy balance, and they are considered as a basic base in the treatment of patients with diabetes. Adequate rest is also very important for maintaining energy levels and wellbeing, and all patients should be advised to sleep approximately 7 hours per night whereas sleep deprivation aggravates insulin resistance, hypertension, hyperglycemia and dyslipidemia.

Pharmacological interventions. Typically, various drug classes can be used to control type 2 diabetes, including human insulin analogs, drugs that reduce insulin resistance (biguanides and thiazolidinediones or glitazones), secretagogues and their analogues (sulfonylureas, meglitinides, inhibitors of dipeptidyl peptidase IV (DPP-4) or agonists and analogues of glucagon-like peptide-1 (GLP-1)), and drugs that reduce the rate of carbohydrate degradation (alpha-glucosidase inhibitors).

Many oral drugs, such as metformin (biguanide), sulfonylureas and thiazolidinediones are often recommended as the first option for the treatment of the disease by the American Diabetes Association (ADA) and European Association for the Study of Diabetes (EASD).

- Gestational diabetes

The primary intervention recommended to women diagnosed with gestational diabetes mellitus is dietary counseling in combination with physical activity and self-monitoring of blood glucose. If these measures are insufficient in terms of achieving optimal glycemic control, subcutaneous insulin therapy is recommended as insulin does not cross the placenta and is therefore considered harmless to the fetus. However, insulin is relatively expensive and difficult to administer. It requires education to ensure a safe administration and it is associated with an increased risk of hypoglycemia and weight gain. The use of safe and effective oral agents may offer advantages over insulin but has not yet been formally approved in all countries. Both metformin and sulfonylurea have been increasingly and safely used in the treatment of gestational diabetes.

Quality of Life

Diabetes can affect the life of those who suffer from it in many ways: emotionally, physically, financially and socially. Recent studies suggest that diabetes is often associated with a range of psychological problems and mental disorders, which not only cause pain but also affect the treatment and course of the disease.

The psychosocial impact of diabetes and its treatment can cause psychological problems and mental disorders, which require psychiatric consultation for the recognition and treatment of its clinical manifestations. Very typical emotional responses to the disease situation are a sense of danger, loss of vital social role performance and loss of opportunities. The condition can cause aggression, defensive reactions appearing as excessive anger, irritability, suspicion and abnegation. It can also result in timid, shy and insecure behavior or maliciousness and suspiciousness.

Prevention

At present, there are no known methods to prevent type 1 diabetes. Research studies have found that lifestyle changes can prevent or delay the onset of type 2 diabetes among high-risk adults or those identified with prediabetes. Lifestyle interventions include diet and moderate-intensity physical activity (such as walking for at least 150 minutes each week). For both sexes and all age and racial and ethnic groups, the development of diabetes was reduced 40%-60% during intensive blood glucose control studies that lasted 3 to 6 years. Studies have also shown that medications such as metformin have been successful in preventing diabetes in some population groups, although to a lesser degree than lifestyle intervention. Lifestyle changes and medications should be combined together to prevent type 2 diabetes.

(Extracted from https://www.ncbi.nlm.nih.gov)

Vocabulary

hyperglycemia	[ˌhaɪpərglaɪˈsiːmɪə]	n. 高血糖（症）
postprandial	[ˌpəʊstˈprændɪəl]	adj. 饭后的；餐后的
subcutaneous	[ˌsʌbkjʊˈteɪnɪəs]	adj. 皮下的
bolus	[ˈbəʊləs]	n. （单次给药的）剂量
basal	[ˈbeɪsl]	adj. 基底的
thiazolidinediones	[θɪætsɒˈlaɪdɪniːdɪəz]	n. 噻唑烷二酮类
secretagogue	[sɪˈkriːtəgɒg]	n. 促分泌素
sulfonylureas	[sʌlfɒnɪˈlʊːrɪəz]	n. 磺脲类
meglitinides	[megˈlaɪtɪnaɪdz]	n. 氯茴苯酸类
biguanides	[bɪgˈwaːnɪdz]	n. 双胍类
peptidase	[ˈpeptɪˌdeɪs]	n. 肽酶
carbohydrate	[ˌkaːrbəʊˈhaɪdreɪt]	n. 碳水化合物；糖类
metformin	[metˈfɔːmɪn]	n. 二甲双胍
fetus	[ˈfiːtəs]	n. 胚胎；胎儿
irritability	[ˌɪrɪtəˈbɪləti]	n. 易怒；过敏性；兴奋性
prediabetes	[ˌpriːdaɪəˈbiːtiːz]	n. 前驱糖尿病
macrosomia	[mækrəʊˈsəʊmɪə]	n. 巨大胎儿；巨体；巨大症

Exercises

1. Read the text and explain the following medical phrases.

1) Clinical characteristics of diabetes

2) Types of diabetes

3) Causes of type 1 diabetes

4) Causes of type 2 diabetes

5) Definition of gestational diabetes

2. Answer the following questions according to the text.

1) What must type 1 diabetes patients do in their daily life?

2) How does a doctor diagnose diabetes?

3) How may gestational diabetes influence the infant?

4) Do you know how to prevent diabetes?

3. Fill in the blanks with the proper forms of the given words.

| socioeconomic | morbidity | disable | controll | therapy |
| obese | hypoglycemia | insulin | microvascular | minimize |

Type 2 diabetes is characterized by relative 1)_____ deficiency and insulin resistance in target organs. Between 1980 and 2004, the global rise in 2)_____, sedentary lifestyles, and an ageing population have quadrupled the incidence and prevalence of type 2 diabetes. As the sixth leading cause of 3)_____ in 2015, diabetes places considerable socioeconomic pressures on the individual and 4)_____ costs to global health economies, estimated at US $825 billion. Cardiovascular disease is the greatest cause of 5)_____ and mortality associated with type 2 diabetes and the patient needs intensive management of glucose and lipid concentrations as well as blood pressure to 6)_____ the risk of complications and disease progression. The benefits of intensive glucose management on 7)_____ complications, such as retinopathy, nephropathy, and neuropathy, have been shown in several large randomized 8)_____ trials.

Evidence that intensive glucose reduction reduces macrovascular outcomes is less well established. Hypoglycemia is a major barrier to optimizing the 9)_____ lowering control, and results of an observational study showed that severe 10)_____ was associated with increased mortality at 12 months even in people not receiving insulin.

4. **Study the bold-faced words in each of the following sentences and imitate the particular way of writing.**

Mentor Sentence：

☆ In morbidly obese patients，bariatric surgery **can be an effective means of** weight loss.

Imitation Sentence：

☆ Parenteral vaccination **can be an effective means of** inducing protective mucosal responses.

1) Diabetes **has remained as the** 5th **leading cause of** death worldwide **and has directly resulted in** 1.6 million deaths.

Answer：_____ **has remained as the** _____ **leading cause of** _____ **and has directly resulted in** _____

_____

2) Urine test and blood tests **are conducted to detect** diabetes **by checking for** excess body glucose.

Answer：_____ **are conducted to detect** _____
by checking for _____

_____

3) Type 1 diabetes **is distinguished by** deficient insulin production in the body.

Answer：_____ **is distinguished by** _____

_____

4) Dietary intake and physical exercise **are the two main determinants of** the energy balance，**and they are considered as** a basic base in the treatment of patients with diabetes.

Answer：_____ **are the two main determinants of** _____，
and they are considered as _____

_____

5. **Match the following statements with the corresponding sections in the text.**

Epidemiology：_____   Management：_____
Mechanisms/Pathophysiology：_____   Quality of Life：_____
Diagnosis：_____   Prevention：_____

A. Diabetes mellitus (DM) is a metabolic disorder resulting from a defect in insulin secretion，insulin action，or both.

B. It is the most common endocrine disorder.

C. By the year 2010，it is estimated that more than 200 million people worldwide will have DM and 300 million will subsequently have the disease by 2025.

D. Diabetes mellitus may be categorized into several types and the two major types are type 1 and type 2.

E. As the disease progresses, tissue or vascular damage ensues leading to severe diabetic complications such as retinopathy, neuropathy, nephropathy, cardiovascular complications and ulceration.

F. Thus, diabetes covers a wide range of heterogeneous diseases.

G. Diabetes mellitus is diagnosed with a test for the glucose content in the blood.

H. Drugs are used primarily to save life and alleviate symptoms.

I. Secondary aims are to prevent long-term diabetic complications and, by eliminating various risk factors, to increase longevity.

J. Insulin replacement therapy is the mainstay for patients with type 1 DM while diet and lifestyle modifications are considered the cornerstone for the treatment and management of type 2 DM.

K. Insulin is also important in type 2 DM when blood glucose levels cannot be controlled by diet, weight loss, exercise, and oral medications.

L. Oral hypoglycemic agents are also useful in the treatment of type 2 DM.

M. Diabetes is best prevented and controlled either by diet alone and exercise (non-pharmacological), or diet with herbal or oral hypoglycemic agents or insulin (pharmacological).

N. Diabetes can affect the life of those who suffer from it in many ways: emotionally, physically, financially and socially.

6. Read the introduction in the box and finish the exercises after it.

> *Order of importance*, *widely used in sciences, especially lab texts and experiments, shows information **from** either **the most important part to the least important part** or vice versa. The writer might begin a paragraph with the supporting detail that "packs the most punch" and end with a weaker idea. The writer can also do the opposite by beginning the paragraph with a less forceful idea and ending it with a stronger one.*

1) Circle the most important information and underline the less important ones.

Diabetes raises the risk of developing high blood pressure, which puts further strain on the patient's heart load. The high blood glucose levels of the patient can provocate the formation of fatty deposits in blood vessel walls. Over time, it can restrict the blood flowing speed and increase the risk of atherosclerosis, or hardening of the blood vessels.

2) Reorder the following sentences to make an effective paragraph.

A. Smoking, elevated cholesterol levels, obesity, high blood pressure, and lack of regular exercise increase the adverse effects of diabetes.

B. People who have well-controlled blood sugar levels show far less common and severe complications of diabetes mellitus.

C. Wider health problems accelerate the deleterious effects of diabetes.

Answer: __ __ __

7. Translate the Chinese paragraph below into English.

糖尿病是由于胰腺不产生或者较少产生胰岛素及机体对胰岛素耐受而引起的疾病。糖尿病可以分为 1 型糖尿病和 2 型糖尿病。大多数糖尿病患者由于遗传和家族史而患有 2 型糖尿病。糖尿病患者应该管理每日饮食摄入量。如果患者正在服用降糖药，但不控制饮食，那么就有可能出现低糖血症，这可能比高血糖症更危险。

8. Read the text and fill in the sheet with proper information.

Reading Prompts	
Items	**Your Answers**
1) Identify the medical terms concerning **diabetes mellitus** and group them according to your understanding.	
2) Identify the **adjectives** used in "**Clinical presentation**" and explain what conditions they describe.	
3) Identify the **conjunctions** used in "**Quality of Life**" part and point out the logical relation each of them indicates.	
4) Identify the **verbs** used in **Exercise 3** and point out the changes of verb tenses.	
5) Identify the **typical sentence patterns.** (**the whole article**)	
6) Identify the **topic sentence** and the **supporting sentences** in "**Prevention**".	

Title: _____

In 1920 Frederick Grant Banting (1891 – 1941) was a surgeon in a floundering practice in London, Ontario, Canada. The youngest son of Methodist farmers from Alliston, Ontario, Banting almost entered the Methodist ministry but decided at the last moment that his calling lay in medicine. World War I shortened his five-year medical course at the University of Toronto: his class did its entire fifth year during the summer of 1916 and, upon receiving their hasty degrees, went off to war. Banting served as a battalion medical officer in the Canadian Army Medical Corps; he returned to Toronto in 1919 after having been wounded in the arm by shrapnel. He, trained as a surgeon at the Hospital of Sick Children in Toronto, then decided to open a small practice as a surgeon in London, Ontario. Unfortunately, his earnings from his practice were meager, forcing him to take a position as a demonstrator in the local medical school. It was in this capacity that Banting was preparing a lecture about the function of the pancreas on October 30, 1920. He stopped at the medical school library, where he picked up the latest issue of Surgery, Gynecology and Obstetrics, and read an article titled "The Relation of the Islets of Langerhans to Diabetes, with Special Reference to Cases of Pancreatic Lithiasis."

While thinking about pancreatic secretions after reading the article, Banting jotted down an idea for a preliminary experiment to further investigate the relationship between pancreatic secretions and diabetes. On November 7, following the advice of a colleague, Banting brought his idea to the attention of John James Rickard Macleod (1876 – 1935), a Scottish physiologist and expert in carbohydrate metabolism at his alma mater, the University of Toronto.

Earlier in his career, Macleod had published a series of papers on glycosuria, or the presence of sugar in the urine (a common indication of diabetes). As a scientist familiar with the literature on the subject, he was unimpressed with Banting's range of knowledge about diabetes and the pancreas and skeptical about the soundness of Banting's idea. However, Macleod decided to give him lab space, an assistant and some laboratory dogs for two months at the end of the academic year.

Banting and his assistant, Charles Herbert Best (1899 – 1978), began their experiments in May 1921. Best, the American son of Canadian parents had just finished his bachelor's degree in physiology and biochemistry at the University of Toronto and had been hired as a research assistant to Macleod, his former teacher. Macleod assigned him to Banting, and the 29-year-old surgeon and the 22-year-old assistant began their work together.

A combination of timing and good luck enabled the Toronto researchers to be the first to announce the discovery of insulin. Scientists in Germany and Hungary had come very close to finding pure insulin, but lack of funding and the devastation of World War I halted their progress. Following in the footsteps of earlier researchers, Banting and Best began to study diabetes through an experimental combination of duct ligation, which involved tying off the pancreatic duct to the small intestine, and pancreatectomies, or the complete surgical removal of the pancreas. Duct ligation served to atrophy the acini cells that produced the digestive secretions, leaving behind only the cells of the islets of Langerhans. Duct-ligated dogs, it was discovered, did not develop diabetes. Pancreatectomy was the method of inducing diabetes: when all pancreatic tissue was removed, the experimental dogs immediately showed signs of glycosuria.

Banting's idea of October 30 involved ligation of the pancreatic ducts of a dog and the extraction and isolation of whatever secretions were produced after the atrophy of the acini cells. He and Best began this experiment, only to find that it was difficult to keep duct-ligated, depancreatized dogs alive long enough to carry out any tests. After a summer of many setbacks and failures, however, the team reported in the fall that they were keeping a severe diabetic dog alive with injections of an extract made from duct-ligated pancreas and prepared, following Macleod's instructions, in saline. Amazingly, this extract dramatically lowered the blood sugar levels of diabetic experimental dogs.

At the end of 1921, Macleod invited James Bertram Collip (1892 – 1965), a biochemist in the department of physiology at the University of Toronto, to help Banting and Best with purifying their extract. As the experimental pace quickened, Banting and Best needed large amounts of their extract, and Collip set to work purifying the extract for clinical testing in humans.

The first clinical tests on a human patient were conducted on a severely diabetic 14-year-old boy. Although the injections of the extract failed to have resoundingly beneficial effects, the Toronto team continued to experiment. A short while later Collip made a breakthrough in purifying the extract, using alcohol in slightly over 90 percent concentration to precipitate out the active ingredient (insulin).

Banting and Macleod received the 1923 Nobel Prize in Physiology or Medicine for the discovery of insulin. By the end of 1923 insulin had been in commercial production for a year at the Eli Lilly and Company laboratories in Indianapolis. Diabetic patients who received insulin shots recovered from comas, resumed eating carbohydrates (in moderation) and realized they had been given a new lease on life.

(Extracted from https://www. sciencehistory. org)

Exercises

1. Read the article and write a possible title for it.

2. Answer the following questions according to the passage.

1) Who was Frederick Grant Banting?

2) What was Banting's idea of October 30?

3) How did Macleod assist Banting?

4) What was the obstacle of Banting and Best's experiment?

5) What breakthrough did Collip make?

UNIT 16 Psychiatry

Psychiatry is a branch of medicine focusing on the diagnosis, treatment and prevention of mental, emotional and behavioral disorders. Mental disorders include depression, bipolar disorder, schizophrenia, dementia, and developmental disorders including autism.

Part I Intensive Reading

Schizophrenia

Schizophrenia is a serious mental illness that affects how a person thinks, feels, and behaves. People with schizophrenia may seem like they have lost touch with reality, which causes significant distress for the individual, their family members and friends. If left untreated, the symptoms of schizophrenia can be persistent and disabling. However, effective treatments are available. When delivered in a timely, coordinated, and sustained manner, treatment can help affected individuals to engage in school or work, achieve independence, and enjoy personal relationships.

Epidemiology

Each year 1 in 10000 adults (12 to 60 years of age) develops schizophrenia. Based on a restrictive and precise definition of the diagnosis and using standardized assessment methods and large, representative populations, the incidence rates appear stable across countries and cultures and over time, at least for the last 50 years. Schizophrenic patients are not born into ecological and social disadvantage. The uneven distribution of prevalence rates is a result of social selection: an early onset leads to social stagnation, and a late onset to descent from a higher social status. The main age range of risk for schizophrenia is 20 to 35 years. It is still unclear whether schizophrenia-like late-onset psychoses (for example, late paraphrenia) after age 60 should be classified as schizophrenia either psychopathologically or etiologically.

In 75% of cases, first admission is preceded by a prodromal phase with a mean length of 5 years and a psychotic prephase of one year's duration. On average, women fall ill 3 to 4 years later than men and show a second peak of onset around menopause. Consequently, late-onset schizophrenias are more frequent and more severe in women than in men. The sex difference in age of onset is smaller in cases with a high genetic load and greater in cases with a low genetic load. Type of onset and core symptoms do not differ between the sexes. The most pronounced sex difference is the socially negative illness behavior of young men.

Mechanisms/Pathophysiology

Schizophrenia is a complex illness. Mental health experts are not sure what causes it. Genes may play a role. Schizophrenia is typically diagnosed in the late teen years to the early thirties and tends to emerge earlier in males (late adolescence to early twenties) than females (early twenties to early thirties). Schizophrenia occurs in just as many men as women. It usually begins in the teen or young adult years, but it may begin later in life. In women, it tends to begin slightly later. Schizophrenia in children usually begins after age 5. Childhood schizophrenia is rare and can be hard to tell apart from other developmental problems.

Research suggests that schizophrenia may have several possible causes as below.

Genetics. Schizophrenia is not caused by just one genetic variation, but a complex interplay of genetics and environmental influences. Heredity does play a strong role—your likelihood of developing schizophrenia is more than six times higher if you have a close relative, such as a parent or sibling, with the disorder.

Environment. Exposure to viruses or malnutrition before birth, particularly in the first and second trimesters has been shown to increase the risk of schizophrenia. Recent research also suggests a relationship between autoimmune disorders and the development of psychosis.

Brain chemistry. Problems with certain brain chemicals, including neurotransmitters called dopamine and glutamate, may contribute to schizophrenia. Neurotransmitters allow brain cells to communicate with each other. Networks of neurons are likely involved as well.

Substance use. Some studies have suggested that taking mind-altering drugs during teen years and young adulthood can increase the risk of schizophrenia. A growing body of evidence indicates that smoking marijuana increases the risk of psychotic incidents and the risk of ongoing psychotic experiences. The younger and more frequent the use, the greater the risk.

Diagnosis

It can be difficult to diagnose schizophrenia in teens. This is because the first signs can include a change of friends, a drop in grades, sleep problems, and irritability—common and nonspecific adolescent behavior. Other factors include isolating oneself and withdrawing from others, an increase in unusual thoughts and suspicions, and a family history of psychosis. In young people who develop schizophrenia, this stage of the disorder is called the "prodromal" period. A diagnosis of schizophrenia often follows the first episode of psychosis, when individuals first display symptoms of schizophrenia. Gradual changes in thinking, mood and social functioning often begin before the first episode of psychosis, usually starting in mid-adolescence. Schizophrenia can occur in younger children, but it is rare for it to occur before late adolescence.

Symptoms usually develop slowly over months or years. The person may have many symptoms, or only a few. People with schizophrenia may have trouble keeping friends and working. They may also have problems with anxiety, depression, and suicidal thoughts or behaviors.

Early symptoms may include:

□ *irritable or tense feelings*

□ *trouble concentrating*

□ *trouble sleeping*

As the illness continues, the person may have problems with thinking, emotions, and behavior including:

□ *hearing or seeing things that are not there (hallucinations)*

□ *isolation*

□ *reduced emotions in tone of voice or expression of face*

□ *problems with understanding and making decisions*

□ *problems with paying attention and following through with activities*

□ *strongly held beliefs that are not real (delusions)*

□ *talking in a way that does not make sense*

With any condition, it is essential to get a comprehensive medical evaluation in order to obtain the best diagnosis. For a diagnosis of schizophrenia, some of the following symptoms are present in the context of reduced functioning for a least 6 months.

Hallucinations. These include a person hearing voices, seeing things, or smelling things that others can't perceive. The hallucination is very real to the person experiencing it, and it may be very confusing for a loved one to witness. The voices in the hallucination can be critical or threatening. Voices may involve people that are known or unknown to the person hearing them.

Delusions. These are false beliefs that do not change even when the person who holds them is presented with new ideas or facts. People who have delusions often also have problems concentrating, confused thinking, or the sense that their thoughts are blocked.

Negative Symptoms. These are ones that diminish a person's abilities. Negative symptoms often include being emotionally flat or speaking in a dull and disconnected way. People with the negative symptoms may be unable to start with or follow through activities, show little interest in life, or sustain relationships. Negative symptoms are sometimes confused with clinical depression.

Cognitive issues/disorganized thinking. People with the cognitive symptoms of schizophrenia often struggle to remember things, organize their thoughts or complete tasks. Commonly, people with schizophrenia have anosognosia or "lack of insight." This means the person is unaware that he has the illness, which can make treating or working with him much more challenging.

Management

During an episode of schizophrenia, the person may need to stay in the hospital for safety reasons. There is no cure for schizophrenia, but it can be treated and managed in several ways.

- Antipsychotic medications

Antipsychotic medications can help reduce the intensity and frequency of psychotic symptoms. They are usually taken daily in pill or liquid forms. Some antipsychotic medications are given as injections once or twice a month, which some individuals find to be more convenient than daily oral doses. Patients whose symptoms do not improve with standard antipsychotic medication typically receive clozapine. People treated with clozapine must undergo routine blood testing to detect a potentially dangerous side effects that occurs in $1\% - 2\%$ of patients.

Many people taking antipsychotic medications have side effects such as weight gain, dry mouth, restlessness and drowsiness when they start taking these medications. Some of these side effects subside over time, but others may persist, which may cause some people to consider stopping their antipsychotic medication. Suddenly stopping medication can be dangerous and it can make schizophrenia symptoms worse. People should not stop taking antipsychotic medication without talking to a health care provider first.

Shared decision making between doctors and patients is the recommended strategy for determining the best type of medication or medication combination and the right dose. The latest information on warnings, patient medication guides, or newly approved medications are on the U. S. Food and Drug Administration (FDA) website.

- Psychosocial treatments

Cognitive behavioral therapy, behavioral skills training, supported employment, and cognitive remediation interventions may help address the negative and cognitive symptoms of schizophrenia. A combination of these therapies and antipsychotic medication is common. Psychosocial treatments can be helpful for teaching and improving coping skills to address the everyday challenges of schizophrenia. They can help people pursue their life goals, such as attending school, working, or forming relationships. Individuals who participate in regular psychosocial treatment are less likely to relapse or be hospitalized.

- Family education and support

Educational programs for family members, significant others, and friends offer instruction about schizophrenia symptoms and treatments, and strategies for assisting the person with the illness. Increasing key supporters' understanding of psychotic symptoms, treatment options, and the course of recovery can lessen their distress, bolster coping and empowerment, and strengthen their capacity to offer effective assistance. Family-based services may be provided on an individual basis or through multi-family workshops and support groups.

- Coordinated specialty care

Coordinated specialty care (CSC) is a general term used to describe recovery-oriented treatment programs for people with first episode psychosis, an early stage of schizophrenia. A team of health professionals and specialists deliver CSC, which includes psychotherapy, medication management, case management, employment and education support, and family education and support. The person with early psychosis and the team work together to make treatment decisions, involving family members as much as possible. Compared to typical care for early psychosis, CSC is more effective at reducing symptoms, improving quality of life, and increasing involvement in work or school.

- Assertive community treatment

Assertive community treatment (ACT) is designed especially for individuals with schizophrenia who are at risk for repeated hospitalizations or homelessness. The key elements of ACT include a multidisciplinary team, including a medication prescriber, a shared caseload among team members, direct service provision by team members, a high frequency of patient contact, low patient to staff ratios, and outreach to patients in the community. ACT reduces hospitalizations and homelessness among individuals with schizophrenia.

Quality of Life

QoL in schizophrenia patients is significantly lower than healthy people, including in physical health, psychological health, social relationships and environmental domains. Clinicians and health authorities should develop effective interventions to address and improve QoL for this population.

Prevention

Antipsychotic drugs are the most effective treatment for schizophrenia. They change the balance of chemicals in the brain and can help control symptoms. These drugs can cause side effects, but many side effects can be managed. Side effects should not prevent the person from being treated for this serious condition.

(Extracted from https://www.nami.org)

Vocabulary

schizophrenia	[ˌskɪtsəˈfriːniə]	n. 精神分裂症
coordinated	[kəʊˈɔːdɪneɪtɪd]	adj. 协调的
psychoses	[saɪˈkəʊsɪs]	n. 精神病；精神不正常
paraphrenia	[ˌpærəˈfriːniə]	n. 妄想痴呆
menopause	[ˈmenəpɔːz]	n. 更年期；活动终止期
heredity	[həˈredəti]	n. 遗传；遗传特征
neurotransmitter	[ˈnjʊərəʊtrænzmɪtə(r)]	n. 神经递质
dopamine	[ˈdəʊpəmiːn]	n. 多巴胺
marijuana	[ˌmærəˈwɑːnə]	n. 大麻
hallucination	[həˌluːsɪˈneɪʃn]	n. 幻觉；幻想
anosognosia	[ənəsɒɡˈnəʊzə]	n. 疾病失认症；病觉缺失
clozapine	[ˈkləʊzəpiːn]	n. 氯氮平
bolster	[ˈbəʊlstə(r)]	v. 支持；鼓励
caseload	[ˈkeɪsləʊd]	n. 待处理案件的数量

Exercises

1. **Read the text and explain the following medical phrases.**

   1) Clinical characteristics of schizophrenia

   2) Causes for schizophrenia

   3) Early Symptoms of schizophrenia

   4) Treatments of schizophrenia

   5) Side effects from antipsychotics

2. **Answer the following questions according to the text.**

   1) What types of individuals are at a high-risk for schizophrenia?

   2) How can we diagnose schizophrenia?

   3) What are the first signs of schizophrenia?

   4) What symptoms may indicate schizophrenia?

3. **Fill in the blanks with the proper forms of the given words.**

affect	smell	hallucination	perception	control
suicide	disorder	schizophrenia	characteristic	psychosis

   Schizophrenia is a brain disorder classified as a 1)_____, which means
   that it affects a person's thinking, sense of self, and 2)_____. The disorder
   typically becomes evident during late adolescence or early adulthood. Signs and
   symptoms of schizophrenia include false perceptions called 3)_____. Auditory
   hallucinations of voices are the most common hallucinations in schizophrenia, but
   4)_____ individuals can also experience hallucinations of visions, 5)_____, or
   touch sensations. Strongly held false beliefs (delusions) are also 6)_____ of
   schizophrenia. For example, affected individuals may be certain that they are a
   particular historical figure or that they are being plotted against or 7)_____ by
   others. People with 8)_____ often have decreased ability to function at school,
   at work, and in social settings. 9)_____ thinking and concentration,
   inappropriate emotional responses, erratic speech and behavior, and difficulty
   with personal hygiene and everyday tasks can also occur. People with
   schizophrenia may have diminished facial expression and animation (flat affect),
   and in some cases become unresponsive. Substance abuse and 10)_____
   thoughts and actions are common in people with schizophrenia. Certain
   movement problems such as tremors, facial tics, rigidity, and unusually slow
   movement (bradykinesia) or an inability to move are common in people with

schizophrenia.

4. Study the bold-faced words in each of the following sentences and imitate the particular way of writing.

Mentor Sentence:

☆ In morbidly obese patients, bariatric surgery **can be an effective means of** weight loss.

Imitation Sentence:

☆ Parenteral vaccination **can be an effective means of** inducing protective mucosal responses.

1) The sex difference in age of onset **is smaller in cases with** a high genetic load and **greater in cases with** a low genetic load.

Answer: _____ **is smaller in cases with** _____
_____ **greater in cases with** _____

2) Schizophrenia **is typically diagnosed in** the late teen years to the early thirties and **tends to emerge earlier in** males (late adolescence to early twenties) **than** females (early twenties to early thirties).

Answer: _____ **is typically diagnosed in** _____
_____ **tends to emerge earlier in** _____
_____ **than** _____

3) **A growing body of evidence indicates that** smoking marijuana **increases the risk of** psychotic incidents and the risk of ongoing psychotic experiences.

Answer: **A growing body of evidence indicates that** _____
_____ **increases the risk of** _____
_____

4) People treated with clozapine **must undergo routine blood testing to** detect a potentially dangerous side effects **that occurs in** $1\%-2\%$ of patients.

Answer: _____ **must undergo routine blood testing to**
_____ **that occurs in** _____
_____

5. Match the following statements with the corresponding sections in the text.

Epidemiology: _____   Management: _____

Mechanisms/Pathophysiology: _____   Quality of Life: _____

Diagnosis: _____   Prevention: _____

A. People with schizophrenia may seem like they have lost touch with reality, which causes significant distress for the individual, their family members and friends.

B. People with the illness can experience employment difficulties, social isolation, poverty, repeated hospitalization, imprisonment, insecure and transient accommodation, homelessness, poor physical health, drug abuse and an increased mortality.

C. When delivered in a timely, coordinated and sustained manner, treatment can help affected individuals to engage in school or work, achieve independence, and enjoy personal relationships.

D. If left untreated, the symptoms of schizophrenia can be persistent and disabling.

E. Schizophrenia is a serious mental illness that affects how a person thinks, feels and behaves.

F. Schizophrenia, a severe mental disorder, is characterized by disturbances in multiple mental modalities, including perception, thinking, self-experience, cognition, affect, volition and behaviors.

G. With the transition from hospital-based care to community-based care, family caregivers play a more important role in the rehabilitation of patients with schizophrenia.

H. It is acknowledged that schizophrenia is a chronic disorder requiring long-term treatment and rehabilitation.

I. Family caregivers take responsibility for providing emotional and economic support, supervising medication intake, maintaining treatment compliance, and promoting social interaction.

6. **Read the introduction in the box and finish the exercises after it.**

> **General to specific pattern** is the most common logical organization used in medical communication. This logical pattern involves the process of moving from a general statement, premise, principle or law to specific details. Medical writers find this logical sequence quite helpful in organizing descriptions of objects and processes, classificatory information, and so on.

1) Single-line the general statement and double-line the specific details.

Many persons with schizophrenia live with their families, and as such family intervention can play an important role in care. Education of patients and families about the nature of schizophrenia and the symptoms of the disease helps them to develop coping strategies, capitalize on their strengths and learn to take better care of oneself. Patients (and their families) treated with family intervention are better able to participate in shared decisional processes. Family psychoeducation offers a valuable opportunity for persons with schizophrenia, their families and healthcare providers to exchange their personal experiences about the disease and its treatment. It is important to highlight that family members can provide a continuity of care for persons with schizophrenia, even if the healthcare operators involved in treatment change over time.

2) Reorder the following sentences to make an effective paragraph.

A. Researchers have also found reduced hippocampal volumes and distinct deformations in the medial and lateral thalamic regions in those with schizoaffective disorder in comparison to controls.

B. Also, white matter abnormalities in multiple areas of the brain, particularly the right lentiform nucleus, left temporal gyrus and right precuneus, are associated with schizophrenia and schizoaffective disorder.

C. The exact pathophysiology of schizoaffective disorder is currently unknown.

D. Some studies have shown that abnormalities in dopamine, norepinephrine and serotonin may play a role.

Answer: __ __ __ __

7. **Translate the Chinese paragraph below into English.**

精神分裂症患者对现实的理解与大多数人不同,他们在思维过程中会产生幻觉、错觉和混乱。虽然目前还没有医学检查能确诊精神分裂症,但常常会发现患者大脑有几个区域的大小与正常人存在差异。据推测这些差异可能是脑组织神经退行性变化的结果。

8. **Read the text and fill in the sheet with proper information.**

Reading Prompts	
Items	**Your Answers**
1) *Identify the medical terms concerning* **schizophrenia** *and group them according to your understanding.*	
2) *Identify the* **adjectives** *used in* "**Mechanisms/Pathophysidogy**" *and explain what conditions they describe.*	

Reading Prompts	
Items	**Your Answers**
3) *Identify the* **conjunctions** *used in* **"Quality of Life"** *and point out the logical relation each of them indicates.*	
4) *Identify the* **verbs** *used in* **Exercise 3** *and point out the changes of verb tenses.*	
5) *Identify the* **typical sentence patterns.** (*the whole article*)	
6) *Identify the* **topic sentence** *and the* **supporting sentences** *in* **"Prevention".**	

Title: _____

Depression is a leading cause of non-fatal disease burden worldwide, with a lifetime prevalence of 9% among European adult men and 17% among European adult women. The economic costs associated with depression are staggering: in 2007, the economic costs of depression alone amounted to €136.3 billion in the European Economic Area. The largest share of these costs stem from reduced productivity (€99.3 billion) and health care costs (€37.0 billion).

At present, European health care systems are not entirely successful in averting depression's disease burden through treatment alone. Given the large number of new cases of depression each year, preventing depression might be a key to sustaining and improving population health.

The onset depressive episode may develop at any moment over the life course. Therefore, it is important that prevention efforts are tailored for particular target groups and age groups. For instance, depression prevention programs need to be available for children and young people during their crucial formative years, young mothers at risk of postpartum depression, and people of working age.

Preventive interventions promote coping and self-management skills among people "at risk" of developing depression. Prevention is likely to offer good value for money, especially when offered as effective, scalable and cost-effective self-help interventions via self-help books, web-based platforms, or via mobile technologies.

It is recommended that depression prevention be integrated in existing health systems. This would require a more comprehensive view from those working in the health care sector, with a focus not only on somatic illnesses, but also on the mental aspects of wellbeing. In addition, it requires a focus not only on the (curative) treatment of acute cases, but also adopting a proactive attitude with regard to early identification of people at risk of developing depression, particularly vulnerable groups. Finally, prevention efforts can and should extend beyond health care settings and be embedded in schools, workplaces and homes for the elderly.

It should be noted that the majority of the reviewed evidence comes from research carried out in West Europe, North America and Australia. This needs to be kept in mind, because the WHO European Region is characterized by a great diversity—economically, demographically, epidemiologically and culturally. Hence, a public health strategy that works well in one country may not offer the best solution in another country.

Overall, the current scientific evidence-base supports preventive action across the countries of the WHO European Region. The task at hand requires substantial investments in preventive mental health care, but the potential benefits can be equally rewarding. After all, mental wellbeing is a key resource for learning, productivity, participation and inclusion.

Substantial efforts are made to make treatments available for depression, however, relatively limited efforts are made to prevent the influx of new cases of depression. According to one Australian study, preventing depression is important because current treatment options can only reduce depression's disease burden by 34%. Similar conclusions were drawn from findings from the WHO European region. These findings show preventive interventions are important in conjunction with evidence-based treatment to decrease the disease burden.

Prevention aims to reduce the risk of becoming depressed by enhancing coping and self-management skills in "at risk" people. Three types of prevention can be distinguished: 1) universal prevention, targeting the general population and promoting resilience and mental fitness; 2) selective prevention directed at people exposed to risk factors; and 3) indicated prevention directed at emerging depressive symptoms not yet meeting the diagnostic criteria for the full-blown disorder promotes self-management. In other words, the distinction between the various types of prevention are made by looking at the target group.

Delivery formats of preventive interventions:

- **Face-to-face contact**

Preventive interventions are most often delivered as face-to-face interventions by trained lay people, nurses, social workers, psychologists or general practitioners.

Interventions can be provided in group or individual format, and tailored to specific groups of people such as a class of pupils, a team of employees, or residents in a nursing home.

Such interventions are typically offered over 4 to 8 sessions of 60 to 90 minutes duration. This way of delivering preventive interventions can be fairly labor-intensive and may not be very cost-efficient in countries where labor is expensive.

- **Self-help tools**

Self-help books and self-help programs that are offered over the Internet (e-health) can be a way to support people in better managing their own health.

Preventive self-help interventions can also be offered digitally through mobile devices such as smart phones and tablets (m-health).

- **Blended interventions**

There is converging evidence that e-health interventions, especially when offered with minimal therapist support, can be as effective as face-to-face interventions offered by qualified therapists.

Blended interventions may offer the best of two worlds: certain parts of the intervention are best guided by a "life" therapist (either face-to-face, by email, or during chat sessions over the Internet), whereas routine aspects of the therapy are perhaps better delegated to the computer.

Economic evidence indicates that depression prevention in adults is cost-effective especially when offered in a self-help format with minimal guidance from a therapist. Preventive e-health interventions are a case in point: they have potential to become cost-effective as they do not rely on scarce resources such as therapists' time but rather promote self-management and are scalable, thus reducing the marginal per-patient costs greatly.

(Extracted from https://www.euro.who.int)

Exercises

1. Read the article and write a possible title for it.

2. Answer the following questions according to the passage.

1) Why was depression an economic burden in Europe by 2007?

2) How can the preventive methods for depression adapt to the health system?

3) What is needed for preventing depression?

4) Do you know how to intervene depression?

5) What will you recommend your community to do to help those with depression or at risk of depression?

UNIT 17 Chinese Medicine

Chinese medicine is formed by summarizing experiences of understanding life, maintaining health, and fighting diseases accumulated in daily life, production and medical practice. Not only does it have systematic theories, but also abundant preventative and therapeutic methods as well.

Part I Intensive Reading

Wind Stroke

Wind stroke is a morbid condition characterized by sudden fainting and loss of consciousness with facial distortion, hemiplegia, and dysphasia, or manifested only as a wry face and hemiplegia.

The differentiating treatments for the disease are referential to hypertensive cerebral hemorrhage, cerebral thrombosis, cerebral embolism, subarachnoid hemorrhage, lacunar cerebral infarction, transient cerebral ischemia, as well as the same symptoms caused by peripheral facial paralysis in Western medicine.

Epidemiology

In traditional Chinese medicine (TCM), this disease is named wind stroke due to its sudden onset, diverse symptoms and rapid changes in conditions, which are remarkably similar to characteristics of the wind. It has a high incidence and mortality rate and often has sequelae. In recent years, the incidence rate has been increasing and the population vulnerable to this disease tends to get younger. Therefore, it is a major disease threatening not only human life but also the quality of life.

For example, stroke in Western medicine, which falls into the category of wind stroke in TCM, has similar incidence and mortality among men and women, but 60% of stroke deaths occur in women. Incidence and mortality are also higher among African Americans than European Americans, with only about two-thirds of this difference accountable by differences in cardiovascular and socioeconomic risk factors. Globally, stroke, as a cause of death, has moved from third to second place in the world and is now the leading cause of physical disability in adults aged 65 years and older.

Mechanisms/Pathophysiology

Deficiency of healthy Qi due to accumulated impairment. Senile decay leads to deficiency of Liver Yin and Kidney Yin, and the hyperactivity of Liver Yang. Or excessive thinking causes deficiency of Qi and Blood, Yin deficiency in the Lower Jiao, hyperactivity of Yang and stirring of wind, upward movement of Qi and Blood to hinder mental activity. As a result, fainting and wind stroke occur.

Intemperance in eating. Intemperance in alcohol, greasy and sweet food, or obese body with Qi deficiency will cause dysfunction of spleen and accumulation of dampness. The accumulation of dampness turns into phlegm-fire. Liver-wind intertwines with phlegm-fire and invades channels and collaterals. This will hinder the consciousness of the patient and wind stroke evokes.

Emotional injury. Overacting of five emotions will cause excessive heart-fire. Usual deficiency of Yin, if intertwined with emotional injury, will cause hyperactivity of Liver Yang, upward adverse flow of Qi and Blood, and mental disorder. As a result, fainting and wind stroke occur.

Attack by pathogenic factors due to Qi deficiency. Given that Qi and Blood are insufficient, wind pathogen will attack channels and collaterals, causing obstruction of Qi and Blood. Given that usual excess of phlegm-dampness is induced by exopathic wind, the channels and collaterals of the patient will be blocked and wind stroke occurs.

Diagnosis

The disease is manifested by acute onset, various causes and changeable conditions with clinical symptoms of sudden fainting accompanied by facial distortion, hemiplegia and dysphasia, or only with a wry face and hemiplegia as its clinical symptoms. Among clinical cases, most cases are caused by endogenous factors, but of course, there are some cases which are aroused by exopathogens. Considering its sudden onset and changeable conditions, like the coming and going of wind, it is named "Zhong Feng" (wind stroke). This is different in meaning from the "Zhong Feng" syndrome mentioned in the *Treatise on Febrile Diseases*, which is the result of Taiyang channel being invaded by pathogenic wind and cold.

Management

The differentiation is based on its degree and urgency. In mild cases, only blood vessels, channels and collaterals are affected but no mental symptoms and pathological changes in Zang and Fu organs happen. In severe cases, Zang-Fu organs are involved and accompanied by mental symptoms.

- Wind stroke involving the channels and collaterals

    1) Deficiency of channels and collaterals, and invasion of the pathogenic wind

    Symptoms: The symptoms include numbness of skin, tingling limbs, sudden distortion of the face, dysphasia, salivation, even hemiplegia, sometimes accompanied with aversion to cold, fever, rigidity of the trunk and arthralgia; thin and whitish tongue coating, and a rapidand floating pulse.

    Main points of differentiation: To differentiate, consider the following points: numbness of the skin, tingling limbs, sudden distortion of the face, dysphasia, sometimes accompanied with symptoms of pathogenic factor attacking the exterior of the body. The patient is in a clear state of mind. This type of wind stoke is common with facial paralysis, transient cerebral ischemia and lacunar cerebral infarction.

    Pathogenesis: Deficiency of healthy Qi and the collaterals and superficial Qi weaken the protective mechanism of the body against diseases. Pathogenic wind invades channels and collaterals and obstructs Qi and Blood.

    Treatment: Expel the wind, nourish the blood and dredge collaterals.

    Recipe: Da Qin Jiu Tang.

    2) Deficiency of Liver Yin and Kidney Yin, and upward invasion of Liver Yang

    Symptoms: The symptoms include usual dizziness and headache, tinnitus and giddiness, insomnia, dreaminess, sudden distortion of the face, rigidity of the tongue and dysphasia, or heavily sluggish limbs, even hemiplegia, red tongue with greasy coating, a wiry, thready and rapid pulse or a wiry and slippery pulse.

    Main points of differentiation: To differentiate, consider the following points like usual dizziness and headache, tinnitus and giddiness, sudden distortion of the face, rigidity of the tongue and dysphasia. The patientis in a clear state of mind. This type of wind stroke is observable in cerebral thrombosis, lacunar cerebral infarction and transient cerebral ischemia.

Pathogenesis: Usual deficiency of Kidney Yin and hyperactivity of Liver Yang causes up-stirring of Wind Yang. The Wind Yang, coercing with phlegm, roams about in channels and collaterals, impeding vessels and collaterals.

Treatment: Nourish Yin, suppresses hyperactive Yang, calms the wind and dredges collaterals.

Recipe: Zhen Gan Xi Feng Tang.

- Wind stroke involving the Zang and Fu organs

This is a case of wind stroke manifested by sudden fainting and loss of consciousness. There are some differences in clinical symptoms between wind stroke block pattern and wind stroke desertion pattern.

1) Wind stroke block pattern

This case is marked by sudden fainting, loss of consciousness, trismus, clenched fists, constipation and dysuria, and spasm of limbs. It can be divided into excessive syndrome of coma with heat syndrome and excessive syndrome of coma with cold manifestations.

2) Excessive syndrome of coma accompanied by heat syndrome

Symptoms: Besides the above symptoms mentioned in the wind stroke block pattern, others include a flushed face, fever, rough breathing, foul breath, restlessness, yellowish and greasy tongue coating, as well as a wiry, slippery and rapid pulse.

Main points of differentiation: Consider sudden fainting, flushed face, fever, trismus, constipation and dysuria, yellowish and greasy tongue coating, as well as a wiry, slippery and rapid pulse. This type is commonly seen in cerebral embolism, hypertensive cerebral hemorrhage and subarachnoid hemorrhage.

Pathogenesis: Hyperactivity of Liver Yang causes wind stirring inside, yang ascending, and upward adverse flow of Qi and Blood. Phlegm mixes with fire and the patient loses his consciousness.

Treatment: Remove heat from the liver, calm the endopathic wind, and induce resuscitation with drugs pungent in flavor and cool in property.

Recipe: Zhi Bao Dan or An Gong Niu Huang Wan.

3) Excessive syndrome of coma with cold manifestations

Symptoms: Besides the above symptoms mentioned in the wind stroke block pattern, there are others as pale complexion with dark lips, lying motionless without dysphoria, cold limbs and profuse sputum and saliva, whitish and greasy tongue coating, as well as a deep, slippery and moderate pulse.

Main points of differentiation: Sudden fainting, trismus, pale complexion with dark lips, unwarm limbs, whitish and greasy tongue coating, as well as a deep, slippery and moderate pulse. This type is often seen in hypertensive cerebral hemorrhage and subarachnoid hemorrhage.

Pathogenesis: Excessive phlegm-dampness is pushed upwards by wind, blocking the seven orifices, and obstructing channels and collaterals internally.

Treatment: Eliminate phlegm, calm the endopathic wind, and induce resuscitation with drugs pungent in flavor and warm in property.

Recipe: Su He Xiang Wan.

4) Wind stroke desertion pattern

Symptoms: The symptoms include sudden fainting, unconsciousness, closed eyes with open mouth, snores, feeble breath, cold limbs with relaxed hands, profuse sweating, incontinence of urine and feces, paralyzed body, flaccid tongue, as well as a thready and weak pulse or a feeble pulse.

Main points of differentiation: Consider sudden fainting, closed eyes with open mouth, cold limbs with relaxed hands, profuse sweating, paralyzed body, incontinence of urine and feces, as well as a feeble pulse. This type is common with hypertensive cerebral hemorrhage and subarachnoid hemorrhage.

Pathogenesis: Upward floating of Yang with Yin fluid exhausted below results in severe exhaustion of healthy Qi and deterioration of consciousness.

Treatment: Supplement Qi to restore Yang and use emergency treatment to rescue patient from perishing of Yang and Yin.

Recipe: Shen Fu Tang plus Sheng Mai San.

Quality of Life

The quality of life of patients with wind stroke depends on whether the patient has a strong body, how strong the healthy Qi is, whether the disease is mild or severe, and whether or not the patient has received proper treatment and nursing in time.

When a patient with wind stroke is rescued from coma, various sequelae will be left with him, such as hemiplegia, dysphasia or distortion of the face, so timely treatment should be given including comprehensive methods like acupuncture and moxibustion, TCM manipulation and massage therapy accompanied with suitable exercises to promote the curative effect.

Quality of life of wind stroke patients was significantly affected physically, mentally and socially. Many patients experience both physical and mental disability following the event. For wind stroke survivors, depression is a common consequence and it is known to be associated with deterioration of quality of life. In fact, stroke morbidity is the leading cause of decreased independence and lowered quality of life among adults. Stroke rehabilitation, however, offers a chance to restore quality of life after a stroke. While damaged brain tissue cannot be healed, stroke recovery techniques can offset some degree of disability. Ideally, rehabilitation helps a patient maintain existing abilities and provides strategies for handling stroke-related disabilities. A need for post-stroke rehabilitation programs with a multidisciplinary team for improving the physical, mental and social quality of life for those patients is mandatory to regain their independent life.

Prevention

The key point to prevent occurrence of wind stroke is to pay more attention to premonitory signs and symptoms and provide active treatment. It is also important to enhance nursing in order to improve the clinical cure rate, reduce comorbidities, and lower the mortality and disability rate. Patients in the acute phase are advised to stay in bed and observe the condition closely. Pay attention to the state of mind, pupils, breath and pulse. If the body temperature exceeds 39℃, cool down the temperature through physical methods and be alert for convulsions, hiccups, hematemesis and collapse. Keep the respiratory tract unobstructed and prevent infection of the lungs, mouth, skin, perineum and other parts. If the patient presents speech disorders like poor speech fluency or muteness, language training is necessary and should be carried out patiently and step by step. After the condition is stable, massage and functional training can be combined. Patients can be guided to exercise themselves to promote recovery of the affected limb function.

(Extracted from *Traditional Chinese International Medicine*)

Vocabulary

distortion	[dɪˈstɔːʃn]	*n*. 变形
hemiplegia	[ˌhemɪˈpliːdʒɪə]	*n*. 偏瘫；半身不遂
dysphasia	[dɪsˈfeɪzɪə]	*n*. 言语障碍症
embolism	[ˈembəlɪzəm]	*n*. 栓塞
subarachnoid	[ˌsʌbəˈræknɒɪd]	*adj*. 蛛网膜下的
lacunar	[ləˈkjuːnə]	*adj*. 陷窝的
sequelae	[sɪˈkwiːliː]	*n*. 后遗症
intemperance	[ɪnˈtempərəns]	*n*. 不节制；酗酒
exopathogen	[ˌeksəˈpæθədʒən]	*n*. 外邪
salivation	[ˌsælɪˈveɪʃn]	*n*. 分泌唾液

arthralgia	[ɑːˈθrældʒə]	n. 关节痛
trismus	[ˈtrɪzməs]	n. 牙关紧闭
dysuria	[dɪsˈjʊərɪə]	n. 排尿困难
spasm	[ˈspæzəm]	n. 痉挛
dysphoria	[dɪsˈfɔːrɪə]	n. 烦躁不安
moxibustion	[ˌmɒksɪˈbʌʃn]	n. 艾灸
convulsion	[kənˈvʌlʃn]	n. 惊厥
hematemesis	[ˌhiːməˈtemɪsɪs]	n. 吐血
perineum	[ˌperɪˈniːəm]	n. 会阴

Exercises

1. Read the text and explain the following medical phrases.

1) Clinical characteristics of wind stroke

2) Mechanisms of wind stroke

3) Differences between mild and severe wind stroke

4) Prevention of wind stroke

2. Answer the following questions according to the text.

1) Why is it named "wind stroke" in TCM?

2) Why is wind stroke a threat for humans?

3) How does emotional injury induce wind stroke?

4) What may affect the QoL for patients with wind stroke?

3. Fill in the blanks with the proper forms of the given words.

> needling   differentiate   suitable   invasion   syndrome
> severe   acupoint   relief   obstruct   progress

    With a course of Bell's palsy within 3 months, the patients with mild facial palsy may be treated with acupuncture and moxibustion, Western drugs, or combined acupuncture and moxibustion with Western drugs, whereas the patients with (1)＿＿＿＿ facial palsy may be treated with acupuncture and moxibustion or combined acupuncture and moxibustion with Western drugs. With a course of more than 3 months, acupuncture and moxibustion treatment is more (2)＿＿＿＿. Acupuncture should be applied as early as possible for Bell's palsy. Acupuncture can control the (3)＿＿＿＿ of the disease, quicken the recovery, and improve the (4)＿＿＿＿ of pain and lacrimation. Bell's palsy is suitably treated according to the stages, (5)＿＿＿＿ and symptoms. In acute and subacute stage, the syndromes involved are mostly（6）_____ of wind-cold or wind-heat. In convalescence and sequela stage, phlegm and blood stasis（7）_____ collaterals, Qi deficiency with blood stasis, and Yin Deficiency producing wind are the main syndromes. The principle of selecting（8）_____ for Bell's palsy is to select local points, points of corresponding meridians and those points according to（9）_____ differentiation. Generally, the points of Yangming meridians are the main ones. The various methods of acupuncture and moxibustion are adopted for Bell's palsy, including filiform（10）_____, moxibustion, electro-acupuncture, etc. Two or more methods are usually used together in clinical practice.

4. **Notice the bold-faced words in each of the following sentences and imitate the particular way of writing.**

Mentor Sentence：

☆ In morbidly obese patients, bariatric surgery **can be an effective means of** weight loss.

Imitation Sentence：

☆ Parenteral vaccination **can be an effective means of** inducing protective mucosal responses.

1）In recent years, **the incidence rate** has been increasing **and the population vulnerable to** this disease tends to get younger.

Answer：_____ **the incidence rate** _____ **and the population vulnerable to** _____

2）**This type is often seen in** hypertensive cerebral hemorrhage and subarachnoid hemorrhage.

Answer：**This type is often seen in** _____

_____

3）This is a case of wind stroke **manifested by** sudden fainting and loss of consciousness.

Answer：_____ **manifested by** _____

_____

4）**The key point to prevent occurrence of** wind stroke **is to** pay more attention to premonitory signs and symptoms and provide active treatment.

Answer：**The key point to prevent occurrence of** _____ __ **is to** _____

5. **Match the following statements with the corresponding sections in the text.**

Epidemiology：_____   Management：_____

Mechanisms/Pathophysiology：_____   Quality of Life：_____

Diagnosis:_____ Prevention:_____

A. Brain injuries resulting from stroke are a major and increasing public health problem in both developed and developing countries worldwide.

B. The TCM equivalent of stroke is a syndrome called "wind stroke", which is characterized by facial paralysis, dysphasia, or aphasia and/or hemiplegia.

C. According to TCM theory, wind stroke is generally the consequence of an inherent defect caused by "internal wind" and "external pathogenic wind".

D. Under certain circumstances, external pathogenic wind, internal wind, "phlegm", "fire", "stagnation" and their interactions may lead to Yin or Qi weakness, "liver fire", "wind-phlegm", "phlegm-dampness", or "blood stasis".

E. The result would be an imbalance between Yin and Yang, disturbance of the blood and Qi circulation, deficiency of Liver Yin and Kidney Yin, stagnation of phlegm and dampness.

F. All these can lead to the sudden onset of wind stroke.

G. The treatment of wind stroke in TCM is aimed at alleviating the patient's symptoms and at eliminating the underlying cause.

H. The basic approach in the treatment of wind stroke takes into account the equilibrium of the relative strength between the patient's body resistance and the intensity of endogenous and exogenous pathogenic factors.

I. The restoration of the patient's resistance and the elimination or weakening of the intensity of pathogenic factors are important.

J. Different prescriptions should be used at different stages of the disease, and further adjusted to suit the individual patient's condition in order to achieve a desirable curative effect.

K. Both basic and clinical research in TCM wind stoke will benefit from increasing international collaborations with Chinese scientists and physicians.

6. **Read the introduction in the box and finish the exercises after it.**

> *Specific-to-general pattern* reverses the one we just discussed. A paragraph written in this pattern begins with the details and leads the reader to the generalization, which may be the thesis or the conclusion.

1) Single-line the general statement and double-line the specific details.

When the body is weakened by an imbalance of Yin and Yang, a weather phenomenon can invade and become a destructive influence. A harmful influence is a natural event that becomes destructive only when the body has an inappropriate relationship with that influence in this state; the body is subjected to a conflict between the injurious influence and Normal Qi. The pernicious influence first invades the Qi Protector. If the Qi Protector is durable, the destructive influence is expelled, and the person recovers. However, if the Qi is weak or the pernicious influence is very strong, an imbalance develops and penetrates deeper, engaging the internal organs more. The imbalances generated by some of the pernicious influences that invade the body are produced suddenly and are characterized by an aversion to the specific influence that generated those imbalances, for example, fear of cold, aversion to wind, fever, chills, body aches and malaise. These symptoms are the result of an attempt to shed the influence that is affecting Normal Qi and the Qi Protector. When a hurtful influence invades the body in this way from the outside, it is called an external pernicious influence.

2) Reorder the following sentences to make an effective paragraph.

A. The superstitious belief that demons travelled with the wind led to the use of words like "Evil Wind Stroke," and this explanation for the causes of the disease has continued to the present.

B. If a person became ill, especially with a sudden onset, that illness may have been attributed to an evil spirit that had entered the person's body.

C. At that time, people believed that the world was full of benevolent spirits and evil spirits, both of which affected human events.

D. In ancient China, people were very concerned with "Wind."

E. In Africa and the Middle East, "zār" is used as a term for malevolent spirits or demons that are thought to possess individuals, mostly women, and cause discomfort or illness.

F. For example, if someone had a stroke or heart attack, an unexpected or severe pain, or loss of consciousness or motor abilities or had died, an evil spirit was thought to have possessed the person's body.

Answer: __ __ __ __ __ __

7. Translate the Chinese paragraph below into English.

脑中风是一组以脑部缺血及出血性损伤症状为主要临床表现的疾病,具有极高的病死率和致残率,主要分为出血性脑中风和缺血性脑中风两大类。脑中风是世界上最重要的致死性疾病之一,主要危险因素包括高血压、糖尿病、心脏病、吸烟、个人或家族病史、年龄等。

8. Read the text and fill in the sheet with proper information.

Reading Prompts	
Items	**Your Answers**
1) *Identify the different causes of* **wind stroke** *and explain them according to your understanding.*	
2) *Identify the* **adjectives** *used in* **"Diagnosis"** *and explain what conditions they describe.*	
3) *Identify the* **conjunctions** *used in* **"Quality of Life"** *part and point out the logical relation each of them indicates.*	
4) *Identify the* **verbs** *used in* **Exercise 3** *and point out the changes of verb tenses.*	
5) *Identify the* **typical sentence patterns**. *(the whole article)*	
6) *Identify the* **topic sentence** *and the* **supporting sentences** *in* **"Prevention".**	

Title: _____

"He who takes medicine and neglects to diet wastes the skills of his doctors." This Chinese proverb highlights one of the key findings of a new study exploring how consumers in China choose between traditional Chinese remedies and Western medicine when seeking treatment.

In "Health Remedies: From Perceptions to Preference to a Healthy Lifestyle," Wharton marketing professor Lisa Bolton, New York University doctoral student Wenbo Wang and Peking University marketing professor Hean Tat Keh looked at how people's perceptions of a given remedy, their perceptions of their illness and other factors influence medical decision making. The researchers also examined how the choice of remedy, be it Western medicine (WM) or traditional Chinese medicine (TCM), impacts the decision to follow a healthy lifestyle.

They found that on the whole, Chinese consumers tend to prefer TCM but will opt for Western medicine in particular situations.

Their study has implications beyond the Chinese market, Bolton and her coauthors note. "Consumers today face a wide array of choice options. Proliferation in choice extends to remedies for illness or disease—including drugs, supplements, radiation, surgery, chiropractic, acupuncture, massage therapy, homeopathy, Ayurveda and TCM, to name a few. In many countries of the world, medical pluralism is the norm, with Western and traditional medicine existing side-by-side in the marketplace. Even in countries with a dominant medical tradition, complementary and alternative medicines are increasingly available," the authors write.

According to Bolton, China is an especially good place to study what influences people's health decisions, because Western medicine and traditional Chinese medicine operate alongside each other there, and both forms of medicine are respected. In fact, she says, people will pick what doctor or hospital to go to depending on whether they are looking for a Western or traditional approach.

"In China, TCM and WM have coexisted for more than 200 years, and both types of medication are licensed as patent medicine and are widely available at pharmacies, hospitals and other outlets," the researchers write.

As a backdrop to their research, Bolton and her coauthors present a basic tutorial on the differences between Western and traditional Chinese medicine. WM "is closely linked to the scientific method and emphasizes empirically measurable biochemical processes that drive disease, its treatment and health," they write, adding that this form of treatment "views all medical phenomena as cause-effect sequences" and relies on drugs, radiation and surgery to alleviate symptoms and cure disease.

"On the other hand, TCM favors a holistic approach, views the universe and body philosophically and develops inductive tools and methods ... to guide restoring the total balance of the body." In Chinese medicine, they add, "the correct balance between Yin and Yang makes up the vital energy, 'Qi', an essential life-sustaining substance of which all things are made."

The researchers analyzed consumer perceptions and preferences by presenting small groups of undergraduate and graduate students in Beijing with various combinations of questions and health scenarios. For instance, for a variety of conditions, the students favored TCM for rheumatoid arthritis and insomnia, and WM for the common cold, coronary heart disease and diarrhea.

Treatment goals and patients' time frames influenced their preferences. "Consumers perceive TCM (versus WM) to have slower action and milder side effects and a greater focus on treating the underlying illness versus alleviating the symptoms," the authors note. Likewise, when consumers were uncertain about their condition and not in any particular hurry for a resolution, they preferred traditional remedies.

In one experiment, they asked participants to read hypothetical scenarios involving a patient's high blood pressure diagnosis and treatment advice based on either a WM or TCM approach.

The researchers found that, in general, WM (versus TCM) "reduces the perceived importance of, and motivation to engage in, complementary health-protective behavior, thereby undermining a healthy lifestyle." In other words, patients taking pills for their high blood pressure may be less apt to see the need to exercise, watch their diet or lose weight.

TCM "is seen as holistic, and when you take a certain kind of medicine you are told specifically what behavior to engage in," she notes.

While the study was done in China, the findings have implications for the U. S. and elsewhere, given the tremendous growth in the popularity of alternative medicine. The authors point out that their research "sheds light on the lay theories of medicine that guide consumer behavior. " Bolton says the study's findings could be important to marketers and advertisers because people also make decisions for themselves about health, and the consumer voice in healthcare decision making is increasing.

"From a consumer perspective, decisions in the health domain are important for individual health and the welfare of society as a whole," the researchers write. "Consumers may be driven by lay theories to make health care choices that do not maximize health outcome—for example, choosing health remedies out of potentially inaccurate perceptions of their action rapidity or treatment focus, or neglecting health protective behaviors when consuming WM (versus TCM). Thus, our findings add to the growing debate on the regulation of health marketing, the role of direct-to-consumer advertising, and marketing efforts to promote a healthy lifestyle. "

(Extracted from https://knowledge_wharton.upenn.edu)

Exercises

1. Read the article and write a possible title for it.

2. Answer the following questions according to the passage.

1) What did Professor Bolton et al. intend to explore in their study?

2) What does the study by Professor Bolton et al. imply?

3) Why is China "an especially good place" for this study?

4) How does TCM differ from Western medicine?

5) When would a patient choose TCM or Western medicine?

Appendix 1　Vocabulary

UNIT 1

exponentially	[ˌekspə'nenʃəlɪ]	*adv.* 成倍地；指数地
epigenetic	[ˌepɪdʒɪ'netɪk]	*adj.* 外成的；后成的
pedigree	['pedɪgriː]	*n.* 家谱；系谱；血统
parenchyma	[pə'reŋkɪmə]	*n.* 实质
senescence	[sɪ'nesns]	*n.* 衰老
oxidative	['ɒksɪdeɪtɪv]	*adj.* 氧化的
rhinovirus	[ˌraɪnəʊ'vaɪərəs]	*n.* 鼻病毒
expectoration	[ɪkˌspektə'reɪʃn]	*n.* 咳痰；吐痰；吐出物
compromise	['kɒmprəmaɪz]	*n.* 损伤
spirometry	[spaɪə'rɒmɪtrɪ]	*n.* 肺活量测定法
auscultation	[ˌɔːskəl'teɪʃn]	*n.* 听诊
rhonchi	['rɒŋkɪ]	*n.* (rhonchus 的复数)干啰音
cyanosis	[ˌsaɪə'nəʊsɪs]	*n.* 紫绀
oximetry	[ɒk'sɪmɪtrɪ]	*n.* 血氧定量法，测氧法
saturation	[ˌsætʃə'reɪʃn]	*n.* 饱和；饱和度；浸透
heterogeneous	[ˌhetərə'dʒiːnɪəs]	*adj.* 异种的；异质的
phenotype	['fiːnətaɪp]	*n.* 显型；表现型
maneuver	[mə'nuːvə]	*n.* 方法
spirometer	[ˌspaɪ'rɒmɪtə]	*n.* 肺活量计
plethysmography	[pliθɪz'mɒgrəfɪ]	*n.* 体积描记术
effusion	[ɪ'fjuːʒn]	*n.* 流出；溢出
interdisciplinary	[ˌɪntə'dɪsəplɪnərɪ]	*adj.* 跨学科的
agonist	['ægənɪst]	*n.* 收缩筋；兴奋剂
muscarinic	[ˌmʌskə'rɪnɪk]	*adj.* 毒蕈碱的
antagonist	[æn'tægənɪst]	*n.* 对抗剂；拮抗剂
anticholinergics	[ˌæntɪˌkɒlɪ'nɜːdʒɪks]	*n.* 抗胆碱能药物
corticosteroid	[ˌkɒːtɪkəʊ'steərɔɪd]	*n.* 皮质类固醇
macrolide	['mækrəlaɪd]	*n.* 大环内酯物
phosphodiesterase	[fɒsfədaɪə'stereɪs]	*n.* 磷酸二酯酶
inhibitor	[ɪn'hɪbɪtə(r)]	*n.* 抑制物

mucolytic	[ˌmjuːkəʊ'lɪtɪk]	*adj*. 黏液溶解的
purulence	['pjʊərʊləns]	*n*. 脓；化脓
amoxicillin	[ə'mɒksɪˌsɪlɪn]	*n*. 阿莫西林
azithromycin	[eɪzɪθrə'maɪsɪn]	*n*. 阿奇霉素
decrement	['dekrɪmənt]	*n*. 渐减；减少
audiometry	[ˌɔːdɪ'ɒmətrɪ]	*n*. 听觉测试法

UNIT 2

preeclampsia	[ˌpriːɪ'klæmpsiːə]	*n*. 先兆子痫
angiogenic	[ˌændʒɪəʊ'dʒenɪk]	*adj*. 生成血管的
eclampsia	[ɪ'klæmpsɪə]	*n*. 子痫
hemoconcentration	[heməkɒnsən'treɪʃn]	*n*. 血浓缩
prostacyclin	[ˌprɒstə'saɪklɪn]	*n*. 环前列腺素
thromboxane	['θrɒm'bɒkseɪn]	*n*. 血栓素
endothelin	[endɒ'θiːlɪn]	*n*. 内皮素
thrombocytopenia	[ˌθrɒmbə(ʊ)ˌsaɪtə(ʊ)'piːnɪə]	*n*. 血小板减少（症）
hemolysis	[hɪ'mɒlɪsɪs]	*n*. 溶血（现象）
glomerular	[glɒ'merʊlə(r)]	*adj*. 肾小球的
vacuolated	['vækjʊəleɪtɪd]	*adj*. 有液泡的
proteinuria	[ˌprəʊtiː'njʊərɪə]	*n*. 蛋白尿
nulliparous	[nʌ'lɪpərəs]	*adj*. 未生育过的
serum	['sɪərəm]	*n*. 血清
creatinine	[kriː'ætəˌniːn]	*n*. 肌酸酐
expectant	[ɪk'spektənt]	*adj*. 怀孕的；待产的
antepartum	[ˌæntɪ'paːtəm]	*adj*. 产前的；分娩前的
intrapartum	[ˌɪntrə'paːtəm]	*adj*. 分娩期的

UNIT 3

calyces	['keɪlɪsiːz]	*n*. 肾盏
pelvis	['pelvɪs]	*n*. 骨盆；肾盂
papillae	[pə'pɪli]	*n*. 乳突
supersaturated	[suːpər'sætʃəreɪtɪd]	*adj*. 过饱和的
propensity	[prə'pensətɪ]	*n*. 倾向；习性
arid	['ærɪd]	*adj*. 干燥的；不毛的
ambient	['æmbɪənt]	*adj*. 周围的；氛围的
idiopathic	[ˌɪdɪə'pæθɪk]	*adj*. 先天的；特发的
jagged	['dʒægɪd]	*adj*. 参差不齐的

oxalate	['ɒksəˌleɪt]	n. 草酸盐
monohydrate	[ˌmɒnəʊ'haɪdreɪt]	n. 一水合物
hypercalciuria	[ˌhaɪpəˌkælsɪ'juːərɪə]	n. 高钙尿
hyperoxaluria	[haɪprɒk'sælʊərɪə]	n. 高草酸尿症
apatite	['æpətaɪt]	n. 磷灰石
dihydrate	[daɪ'haɪdreɪt]	n. 二水合物
tricalcium	[traɪ'kælsɪəm]	n. 三钙
acidic	[ə'sɪdɪk]	adj. 酸的;酸性的
nephrolithiasis	[ˌnefrəʊlɪ'θaɪəsɪs]	n. 肾石病
hyperuricosuria	[haɪprʊərɪ'kəʊsjuːrɪə]	n. 高尿酸尿
struvite	['struːvaɪt]	n. 鸟粪石
ammonia	[ə'məʊnɪə]	n. 氨
urease	['jʊərɪeɪs]	n. 脲酶;尿素酶
colic	['kɒlɪk]	n. 腹胶痛
hyperparathyroidism	[haɪpəpærə'θaɪrɒɪdɪzəm]	n. 甲状旁腺功能亢进
bariatric	[ˌbærɪ'ætrɪk]	adj. 肥胖病治疗学的
radio-opaque	['reɪdiːəʊəʊp'eɪk]	adj. 射线透不过的
radiolucent	['reɪdɪəʊ'luːsnt]	adj. 射线可透过的
urogram	[ərəg'ræm]	n. 尿路造影照片
tomography	[tə'mɒgrəfi]	n. X线断层摄影术
lithotomy	[lɪ'θɒtəmɪ]	n. 切石术
lithotripsy	['lɪθəʊˌtrɪpsi]	n. 碎石术
ureteroscopy	[jʊəriːtə'rəskəpɪ]	n. 输尿管镜检查术
hydronephrosis	[ˌhaɪdrəʊnɪ'frəʊsɪs]	n. 肾盂积水
opioid	[əʊ'piːɒɪd]	n. 类鸦片
paracetamol	[ˌpærə'siːtəmɒl]	n. 扑热息痛
expulsive	[ɪk'spʌlsɪv]	adj. 逐出的
uricosuria	[jʊːrɪ'kəʊsjuːrɪə]	n. 尿酸尿
allopurinol	[æləʊ'pjʊərɪnɒl]	n. 别嘌呤醇
chemolysis	[kɪ'mɒləsɪs]	n. 化学溶蚀
mercaptopropionyl	[mɜːkæptɒprəʊpa'ɪɒnɪl]	n. 巯丙酰
glycine	['glaɪsiːn]	n. 甘氨酸;氨基乙酸
alkalization	[ælkəlaɪ'zeɪʃən]	n. 碱性化
hemiacidrin	[hiːmiːæ'sɪdrɪn]	n. 溶肾石酸素
sulfur	['sʌlfə(r)]	n. 硫(磺)

UNIT 4

mycobacterium	[ˌmaɪkəʊbæk'tɪərɪəm]	*n.* 分枝杆菌
alveolar	[æl'viːələ(r)]	*adj.* 肺泡的；齿槽的
cytokine	['saɪtəʊˌkaɪn]	*n.* 细胞因子
neutrophil	['njʊːtrəˌfɪl]	*n.* 嗜中性粒细胞
necrosis	[ne'krəʊsɪs]	*n.* 坏死；坏疽
hematogenous	[ˌhemə'tɒdʒɪnəs]	*adj.* 造血的
eradication	[ɪˌrædɪ'keɪʃn]	*n.* 消灭，扑灭；根除
miliary	[mɪlɪˌerɪ]	*adj.* 粟粒状的；粟粒大的
sterile	['steraɪl]	*adj.* 不育的；无菌的
regimen	['redʒɪmən]	*n.* 养生法；生活规则
smear	[smɪə(r)]	*n.* 涂片
nodular	['nɒdjʊlə(r)]	*adj.* 结节状的
granulomatous	[ˌgrænjʊ'ləʊmətəs]	*adj.* 肉芽肿的
tubercle	['tjʊːbəkl]	*n.* 结节，小瘤
lymphadenopathy	[lɪmˌfædɪ'nɒpəθɪ]	*n.* 淋巴结病
bacilli	[bə'sɪlaɪ]	*n.* 杆菌（bacillus 的复数）
meningitis	[ˌmenɪn'dʒaɪtɪs]	*n.* 脑膜炎
apices	['eɪpɪsiːz]	*n.* 顶端（apex 的复数）
caseation	[ˌkeɪsɪ'eɪʃ(ə)n]	*n.* 干酪样变；干酪化
pyuria	[paɪ'jʊərɪə]	*n.* 脓尿
isoniazid	[ˌaɪsəʊ'naɪəzɪd]	*n.* 异烟肼（抗结核药）

UNIT 5

appendix	[ə'pendɪks]	*n.* 阑尾
cecum	['siːkəm]	*n.* 盲肠
confluence	['kɒnflʊəns]	*n.* 聚集；合并
hyperplasia	[ˌhaɪpə'pleɪʒə]	*n.* 增生；畸形生长
distension	[dɪ'stenʃn]	*n.* 膨胀，扩张
ulceration	[ˌʌlsə'reɪʃn]	*n.* 溃疡形成
anamnesis	[ˌænæm'nɪsɪs]	*n.* 既往症
retrocecal	[ˌretrəʊ'sɪkəl]	*adj.* 盲肠后的
retroileal	[riːtrɔɪ'liːl]	*adj.* 回肠后位
umbilical	[ʌm'bɪlɪkl]	*adj.* 脐带的
colicky	['kɒlɪkɪ]	*adj.* 疝气痛的；腹绞痛的
constipation	[ˌkɒnstɪ'peɪʃn]	*n.* 便秘

pyrexia	[paɪˈreksɪə]	n.	发热;热病
tachycardia	[ˌtækɪˈkɑːdɪə]	n.	心动过速
resuscitation	[rɪˌsʌsɪˈteɪʃn]	n.	复苏
prophylactic	[ˌprɒfəˈlæktɪk]	adj.	预防性的
		n.	预防性药物
peritonitis	[ˌperɪtəˈnaɪtɪs]	n.	腹膜炎
leukocytosis	[ˌluːkəʊsaɪˈtəʊsɪs]	n.	白细胞增多
laparoscopic	[ˌlæpərəˈskɒpɪk]	adj.	腹腔镜检查的
absces	[ˈæbses]	n.	脓肿;脓疮

UNIT 6

anovulation	[æˌnɒvjʊˈleɪʃn]	n.	排卵停止
acne	[ˈæknɪ]	n.	痤疮
hyperandrogenism	[haɪpəˈrændrɒdʒɪnɪzəm]	n.	雄性激素过多症
hirsutism	[ˈhɜːsjʊˌtɪzəm]	n.	多毛症
oligogenic	[ɒlɪgəˈdʒenɪk]	adj.	寡基因的
androgen	[ˈændrədʒən]	n.	雄激素
ovulatory	[ˈɒvjʊlətərɪ]	adj.	排卵的
intrauterine	[ˌɪntrəˈjuːtəraɪn]	adj.	子宫内的
testosterone	[teˈstɒstərəʊn]	n.	睾酮
menstrual	[ˈmenstrʊəl]	adj.	月经的
globulin	[ˈglɒbjʊlɪn]	n.	球蛋白
gestational	[dʒeˈsteɪʃənəl]	adj.	妊娠期的
glucose	[ˈgluːkəʊs]	n.	葡萄糖
adipose	[ˈædɪpəʊs]	adj.	用于贮存脂肪的
aberrant	[æˈberənt]	adj.	异常的
contraceptive	[ˌkɒntrəˈseptɪv]	n.	避孕药
progestin	[prəʊˈdʒestɪn]	n.	黄体酮
venous	[ˈviːnəs]	adj.	静脉的

UNIT 7

skewed	[skjuːd]	adj.	斜交的,歪斜的
amyloid	[ˈæmɪˌlɔɪd]	adj.	类淀粉的
neurofibrillary	[ˌnjʊərəˈfaɪbrɪlerɪ]	n.	神经原纤维
hyperphosphorylated	[haɪpəfɒsfərɪˈleɪtɪd]	adj.	过度磷酸化的
tau	[tɔː]	n.	蛋白
synaptic	[sɪˈnæptɪk]	adj.	突触的

alteration	[ˌɔ:ltə'reɪʃn]	n.	改变，变更
hippocampus	[ˌhɪpə'kæmpəs]	n.	海马
oligomer	[ə'lɪgəmə]	n.	低聚体
fibril	['faɪbrɪl]	n.	纤维；原纤维
glutamate	['glʊːtəmeɪt]	n.	谷氨酸盐，谷氨酸酯
mitochondrial	[ˌmaɪtəʊ'kɒndrɪəl]	adj.	线粒体的
lysosomal	[ˌlaɪsə'səʊməl]	n.	溶酶体
aggregation	[ˌægrɪ'geɪʃn]	n.	集合；聚合
apathy	['æpəθɪ]	n.	冷漠
atherosclerosis	[ˌæθərəʊsklɪ'rəʊsɪs]	n.	动脉粥样硬化
hydrocephalus	[ˌhaɪdrəʊ'sefələs]	n.	脑水肿，脑积水
cholinesterase	[kəʊlə'nestəreɪs]	n.	胆碱酯酶
cholinergic	[ˌkəʊlɪ'nɜːdʒɪk]	adj.	胆碱(功)能的
acetylcholine	[ˌæsɪtɪl'kɒliːn]	n.	乙酰胆碱
agitation	[ˌædʒɪ'teɪʃn]	n.	激动
neuropsychiatric	[njʊərəʊsaɪ'kɪætrɪk]	adj.	神经精神病学的
prodromal	['prəʊdrəʊməl]	adj.	前驱症状的
hydrogenated	[haɪ'drɒdʒəneɪtɪd]	adj.	氢化的
legume	['legjʊːm]	n.	豆类，豆荚
fortified	['fɔːtɪfaɪd]	adj.	加强的
aerobic	[eə'rəʊbɪk]	adj.	有氧的

UNIT 8

fermentation	[ˌfɜːrmen'teɪʃn]	n.	发酵
biofilm	[ˌbaɪəʊ'fɪlm]	n.	生物膜
cariogenic	[ˌkeərɪə'dʒenɪk]	adj.	生龋齿的
sucrose	['sʊːkrəʊz]	n.	蔗糖
lactic	['læktɪk]	adj.	乳(汁)的
hydroxyapatite	[haɪdrɒksɪ'æpətaɪt]	n.	羟磷灰石
polymorphism	[ˌpɒlɪ'mɔːfɪzəm]	n.	多型现象；多态性
demineralization	[demɪnərəlaɪ'zeɪʃn]	n.	脱盐；脱矿质作用
enamel	[ɪ'næml]	n.	珐琅质；釉质
dilution	[daɪ'lʊːʃn]	n.	稀释物，冲淡物
translucent	[trænz'lʊːsənt]	adj.	半透明的
dentine	['dentiːn]	n.	牙质；牙本质；齿质
proteolytic	[ˌprəʊtɪə'lɪtɪk]	adj.	蛋白质分解的

cementum	[sɪˈmentəm]	n. 牙骨质
interproximal	[ˌɪntəˈprɒksɪməl]	adj. 邻间的
		n. 牙间齐整器
hypoplasia	[ˌhaɪpəˈpleɪʒə]	n. 发育不全
porcelain	[ˈpɔːrsəlɪn]	n. 瓷；瓷器

UNIT 9

neonatal	[ˌniːəʊˈneɪtl]	adj. 新生的；初生的
jaundice	[ˈdʒɔːndɪs]	n. 黄疸
hyperbilirubinemia	[haɪpɜˌbɪliːrʌbaɪˈniːmɪə]	n. 高胆红素血；血胆红素过多
sequela	[sɪˈkwiːlə]	n. 后遗症；并发症
hydration	[haɪˈdreɪʃn]	n. 水合作用
polycythemia	[ˌpɒlɪsaɪˈθiːmjə]	n. 红血球增多症
hydrops	[ˈhaɪdrɒps]	n. 积水
purpura	[ˈpɜːpjʊrə]	n. 紫癜
bruising	[ˈbruːzɪŋ]	n. 挫伤的
syphilis	[ˈsɪfɪlɪs]	n. 梅毒
serology	[sɪəˈrɒlədʒɪ]	n. 血清学
galactosemia	[ɡəlæktəˈsiːmɪə]	n. 半乳糖血症
hepatomegaly	[hepətəʊˈmeɡəlɪ]	n. 肝肿大
urinalysis	[ˌjʊərɪˈnælɪsɪs]	n. 验尿
reticulocyte	[rɪˈtɪkjʊləˌsaɪt]	n. 网状细胞
cholestatic	[kɒlsˈtətɪk]	adj. 胆汁阻塞的；胆汁郁积的
biliary atresia		胆管闭锁
aminoacidemia	[æmɪnəʊˈsaɪdiːmɪə]	n. 氨基酸血症
sepsis	[ˈsepsɪs]	n. 败血症
hypopituitarism	[ˌhaɪpəʊpɪˈtjuːɪtərɪzəm]	n. 垂体机能减退
immunoglobulin	[ˌɪmjʊnəʊˈɡlɒbjʊlɪn]	n. 免疫球蛋白
bilifuscin	[bɪlɪˈfʊsɪn]	n. 胆褐素
isoimmunization	[aɪsəʊɪmjʊnaɪˈzeɪʃn]	n. 同种免疫
encephalopathy	[enˌsefəˈlɒpəθɪ]	n. 脑病
transcutaneous	[ˌtrænzkjʊˈteɪnɪəs]	adj. 经皮的

UNIT 10

atherosclerotic	[ˌæθərəʊskləˈrɒtɪk]	adj. 动脉粥样硬化的
ischemic	[ɪsˈkimɪk]	adj. 局部缺血的
myocardial	[ˌmaɪəˈkɑːdɪəl]	adj. 心肌的

infarction	[ɪnˈfɑːkʃn]	n. 梗塞形成；梗死形成
angina pectoris		心绞痛
glycemic	[glɪˈsemɪk]	adj. 血糖的
thrombosis	[θrɒmˈbəʊsɪs]	n. 血栓症
subendothelial	[sʌbendɒˈθiːlɪəl]	adj. 内皮下的
endothelial	[ˌendəʊˈθiːlɪəl]	adj. 内皮的
cardiorespiratory	[ˌkɑːdɪəʊrɪsˈpaɪərətərɪ]	adj. 心肺的
aneurysm	[ˈænjərɪzəm]	n. 动脉瘤
vasodilator	[ˌvezəʊdaɪˈleɪtə]	n. 血管扩张神经
palpitation	[ˌpælpɪˈteɪʃən]	n. 心悸
ventricular	[venˈtrɪkjʊlə(r)]	adj. 心室的；膨胀的
hypertrophy	[haɪˈpɜːtrəfɪ]	n. 肥大；过度生长
extrasystole	[ˌekstrəˈsɪstəliː]	n. 期前收缩；额外收缩
fascicular	[fəˈsɪkjʊlə(r)]	adj. 成束的
versatility	[ˌvɜːsəˈtɪlətɪ]	n. 多功能性
radioisotope	[ˌreɪdɪəʊˈaɪsətəʊp]	n. 放射性同位元素
angioplasty	[ˈændʒɪəʊplæstɪ]	n. 血管成形术
transluminal	[trænsˈlʊːmɪnəl]	adj. 穿过(血管)腔壁的
nitrate	[ˈnaɪtreɪt]	n. 硝酸盐
prodrug	[ˈprəʊˌdrʌg]	n. 前药
hemodynamic	[ˌheməedaɪˈnæmɪk]	adj. 血液动力学的
vasodilation	[ˌveɪzəʊdaɪˈleɪʃn]	n. 血管舒张
dyslipidemia	[dɪslɪpɪˈdemɪə]	n. 血脂障碍

UNIT 11

putative	[ˈpjuːtətɪv]	adj. 推定的，认定的，公认的
visceral	[ˈvɪsərəl]	adj. 内脏的
dysregulation	[dɪsregjʊˈleɪʃn]	n. 调节障碍，调节异常
comorbidity	[kəʊmɒrˈbɪdətɪ]	n. 疾病；伴随疾病
hydroxytryptamine	[haɪˌdrɒksɪˈtrɪptəmiːn]	n. 羟色胺
nociceptor	[ˌnəʊsɪˈseptə(r)]	n. 伤害感受器，疼痛感受器
myenteric	[ˌmaɪenˈterɪk]	adj. 肠肌层的
plexus	[ˈpleksəs]	n. 神经丛
afferent	[ˈæfərənt]	adj. 传入的；输入的
lactose	[ˈlæktəʊz]	n. 乳糖
malabsorption	[mæləbˈsɒrpʃən]	n. 吸收不良；吸收障碍

microbiota	[maɪkrəʊbaɪˈəʊtə]	n. 小型生物群
migratory	[ˈmaɪɡrətrɪ]	adj. 迁移的
distention	[dɪsˈtenʃən]	n. 膨胀，扩张
sedimentation	[sedɪmenˈteɪʃn]	n. 沉淀
sigmoidoscopy	[ˌsɪɡmɒɪˈdɒskəpɪ]	n. 乙状结肠镜检查
celiac	[ˈsiːlɪæk]	adj. 腹的；腹腔的
sprue	[spruː]	n. 口炎性腹泻

UNIT 12

refractive	[rɪˈfræktɪv]	adj. 屈光
retinopathy	[retɪˈnɒpəθɪ]	n. 视网膜病
corneal	[ˈkɔːnɪəl]	adj. 角膜的
retina	[ˈretɪnə]	n. 视网膜
postnatal	[ˌpəʊstˈneɪtl]	adj. 出生后的；初生婴儿的
emmetropia	[ˌeməˈtrəʊpɪə]	n. 屈光正常；正视眼
hyperopia	[ˌhaɪpəˈrəʊpɪə]	n. 远视
spherical	[ˈsferɪkl]	adj. 球状的
monozygotic	[ˌmɒnəʊzaɪˈɡɒtɪk]	adj. 同卵（的）
dizygotic	[ˌdaɪzaɪˈɡɒtɪk]	adj. 异卵的
diopter	[daɪˈɒptə(r)]	n. （透镜的）屈光度
diverge	[daɪˈvɜːdʒ]	v. 发散；分岔；分开
meridian	[məˈrɪdɪən]	n. 子午线；经线
squint	[skwɪnt]	n. 斜视
scleral	[skˈlerəl]	adj. 巩膜的
congenital	[kənˈdʒenɪtl]	adj. 先天的；天生的
macular	[ˈmækjʊlə]	adj. 有斑点的；（眼球）黄斑的
glaucoma	[ɡlɔːˈkəʊmə(r)]	n. 青光眼
peripheral	[pəˈrɪfərəl]	adj. 周围的；外围（的）
lattice	[ˈlætɪs]	n. 格栅；斜条结构
optometry	[ɒpˈtɒmətrɪ]	n. 验光；视力测定
retinoscope	[ˈretənəˌskəʊp]	n. 视网膜镜
curvature	[ˈkɜːvətʃər]	n. 曲率；弯曲；曲度
intraocular	[ˌɪntrəˈɒkjʊlə(r)]	adj. 眼内的
bifocals	[ˌbaɪˈfəʊklz]	n. 双光眼镜

UNIT 13

| epithelium | [ˌepɪˈθiːlɪəm] | n. 上皮；上皮细胞 |

lobular	[ˈlɒbjʊlər]	adj. 有小叶的;有小裂片的
aberration	[ˌæbəˈreɪʃn]	n. 异常
sarcoma	[sɑːˈkəʊmə]	n. 肉瘤,恶性毒瘤
lymphoma	[lɪmˈfəʊmə]	n. 淋巴瘤
proliferative	[prəˈlɪfəˌreɪtɪv]	adj. 增殖的;增生的
menarche	[meˈnɑːkɪ]	n. 初潮
menopausal	[ˌmenəˈpɔːzl]	adj. 绝经期的;更年期的
malaise	[məˈleɪz]	n. 不适
asymmetry	[ˌeɪˈsɪmətrɪ]	n. 不对称
dimpling	[ˈdɪmplɪŋ]	adj. 坑坑洼洼
erythema	[ˌerɪˈθiːmə]	n. 红斑;红疹
cervical	[səˈvaɪkl]	adj. 颈部的
palpate	[pælˈpeɪt]	v. 触诊
adenopathy	[ˌædɪˈnɒpəθɪ]	n. 淋巴结肿大
subareolar	[sʌbeəˈrɪələ]	adj. 乳晕下的
mammography	[mæˈmɒgrəfɪ]	n. 乳房 X 线照相术
metastases	[məˈtæstəsɪːz]	n. 转移
axillary	[ˈæksɪlərɪ]	adj. 腋窝的
scleroderma	[ˌsklɪərəˈdɜːmə]	n. 硬皮病
ipsilateral	[ˌɪpsɪˈlæt(ə)r(ə)l]	adj. 身体同侧的
mastectomy	[mæsˈtektəmɪ]	n. 乳房切除术
sentinel	[ˈsentɪnl]	n. 前哨
lumpectomy	[lʌmˈpektəmɪ]	n. 乳房肿瘤切除术

UNIT 14

aerosol	[ˈerəsɔːl]	n. 气溶胶
angiotensin	[ˌændʒɪəʊˈtensən]	n. 血管紧缩素
convalescent	[ˌkɒnvəˈlesənt]	adj. 恢复期的
desquamation	[ˌdeskwəˈmeɪʃən]	n. 脱屑;脱皮
disproportionate	[ˌdɪsprəˈpɔːrʃənət]	adj. 不成比例的
disseminate	[dɪˈsemɪneɪt]	v. 散播
endotracheal	[ˌendəʊˈtreɪkɪəl]	adj. 气管内的
fibrosis	[faɪˈbrəʊsɪs]	n. 纤维症
glycyrrhizin	[glɪˈkɜːraɪzɪn]	n. 甘草素
haplotype	[ˈhæpləʊtaɪp]	n. 单倍体
hyaline	[ˈhaɪəlɪn]	adj. 透明的

pegylated	['piːdʒɪleɪtɪd]	adj. 加入聚乙二醇的
peptide	['peptaɪd]	n. 肽
placebo	[plə'siːbəʊ]	n. 安慰剂
recombinant	[riː'kɒmbənənt]	n. 重组细胞
specimen	['spesɪmən]	n. 标本;样本
viremia	[vaɪ'riːmɪə]	n. 病毒血症

UNIT 15

hyperglycemia	[ˌhaɪpərglaɪ'siːmɪə]	n. 高血糖(症)
postprandial	[ˌpəʊst'prændɪəl]	adj. 饭后的;餐后的
subcutaneous	[ˌsʌbkjuː'teɪnɪəs]	adj. 皮下的
bolus	['bəʊləs]	n. (单次给药的)剂量
basal	['beɪsl]	adj. 基底的
thiazolidinediones	[θɪætsɒ'laɪdɪniːdɪəz]	n. 噻唑烷二酮类
secretagogue	[sɪ'kriːtəgɒg]	n. 促分泌素
sulfonylureas	[sʌlfɒnɪ'lʊːrɪəz]	n. 磺脲类
meglitinides	[meg'laɪtɪnaɪdz]	n. 氯茴苯酸类
biguanides	[bɪg'waɪnɪdz]	n. 双胍类
peptidase	['peptɪˌdeɪs]	n. 肽酶
carbohydrate	[ˌkaːrbəʊ'haɪdreɪt]	n. 碳水化合物;糖类
metformin	[met'fɔːmɪn]	n. 二甲双胍
fetus	['fiːtəs]	n. 胚胎;胎儿
irritability	[ˌɪrɪtə'bɪlətɪ]	n. 易怒;过敏性;兴奋性
prediabetes	[ˌpriːdaɪə'biːtiːz]	n. 前驱糖尿病
macrosomia	[mækrəʊ'səʊmɪə]	n. 巨大胎儿;巨体;巨大症

UNIT 16

schizophrenia	[ˌskɪtsə'friːnɪə]	n. 精神分裂症
coordinated	[kəʊ'ɔːdɪneɪtɪd]	adj. 协调的
psychoses	[saɪ'kəʊsɪs]	n. 精神病;精神不正常
paraphrenia	[ˌpærə'friːnɪə]	n. 妄想痴呆
menopause	['menəpɔːz]	n. 更年期;活动终止期
heredity	[hə'redətɪ]	n. 遗传;遗传特征
neurotransmitter	['njʊərəʊtrænzmɪtə(r)]	n. 神经递质
dopamine	['dəʊpəmiːn]	n. 多巴胺
marijuana	[ˌmærə'waːnə]	n. 大麻
hallucination	[həˌluːsɪ'neɪʃn]	n. 幻觉;幻想

anosognosia	[ənəsɒgˈnəʊzə]	*n.* 疾病失认症,病觉缺失	
clozapine	[ˈkləʊzəpiːn]	*n.* 氯氮平	
bolster	[ˈbəʊlstə(r)]	*v.* 支持;鼓励	
caseload	[ˈkeɪsləʊd]	*n.* 待处理案件的数量	

UNIT 17

distortion	[dɪˈstɔːʃn]	*n.* 变形
hemiplegia	[ˌhemɪˈpliːdʒɪə]	*n.* 偏瘫;半身不遂
dysphasia	[dɪsˈfeɪzɪə]	*n.* 言语障碍症
embolism	[ˈembəlɪzəm]	*n.* 栓塞
subarachnoid	[ˌsʌbəˈræknɒɪd]	*adj.* 蛛网膜下的
lacunar	[ləˈkjuːnə]	*adj.* 陷窝的
sequelae	[sɪˈkwiːliː]	*n.* 后遗症
intemperance	[ɪnˈtempərəns]	*n.* 不节制;酗酒
exopathogen	[ˌeksəˈpæθədʒən]	*n.* 外邪
salivation	[ˌsælɪˈveɪʃn]	*n.* 分泌唾液
arthralgia	[aːˈθrældʒə]	*n.* 关节痛
trismus	[ˈtrɪzməs]	*n.* 牙关紧闭
dysuria	[dɪsˈjʊərɪə]	*n.* 排尿困难
spasm	[ˈspæzəm]	*n.* 痉挛
dysphoria	[dɪsˈfɔːrɪə]	*n.* 烦躁不安
moxibustion	[ˌmɒksɪˈbʌsʃn]	*n.* 艾灸
convulsion	[kənˈvʌlʃn]	*n.* 惊厥
hematemesis	[ˌhiːməˈtemɪsɪs]	*n.* 吐血
perineum	[ˌperɪˈniːəm]	*n.* 会阴

Appendix 2　Preview Summary

Class number:_____　　　　**Unit**:_____　　　　**Date**:_____

Class comment:			
Review Table	**Exercise 1**	Good ones Examples: Comments:	Poor ones Examples: Comments:
	Exercise 2	Good ones Examples: Comments:	Poor ones Examples: Comments:
	...		
	Advices:		
Special Points:			

Appendix 3　Medical Topics of Ethics

Number	Medical Topics of Ethics
1	Socratic oath
2	Adaption to the heavy study of medical courses
3	Qualities to be a good doctor
4	Stories in fighting pandemics
5	History of hospitals
6	Adaption to the hospital job
7	Safety of medical staff
8	Medical costs
9	Income of doctors
10	Children care
11	Maternal care
12	Senile care
13	Relationships between doctor and patient
14	Doctor education
15	Effective inquire
16	Ethical problems concerning surrogacy
17	HIV patients care
18	Dignity of patients
19	Death education and palliative care
20	Public health education
21	Differences between Western medicine and TCM

Acknowledgement

For this textbook, I specially devote my thanks to Professor Bai Yongquan and Vice Professor Nie Wenxin of Xi'an Jiaotong University. I also want to send my special thanks to all the authors of the original medical articles. I also want to say a small thanks to my daughter, Li Wenqing, who has double check the questions in the exercises. I also want to thank the foreign teacher of our school, Miss Susannah Hazel Boyce who has proofread the whole chapters. I also want to thank the Dean and Vice Dean of my university, Chen Xiangjing and Li Ying for all their support. Finally, I want to send my heartfelt thanks to all those that I have not mentioned here but actually have been very helpful for the publication of this book.